NATURAL HEALING SECRETS

AN A-TO-Z GUIDE TO
THE BEST HOME REMEDIES

FOREWORD BY
DIAN DINCIN BUCHMAN, Ph.D.

BRIAN CHICHESTER

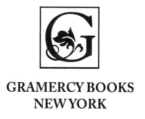

GRAMERCY BOOKS
NEW YORK

This 1998 edition is published by Gramercy Books,®
a division of Random House Value Publishing, Inc.,
201 E. 50th Street, New York, NY 10022,
under arrangement with Ottenheimer Publishers, Inc.
5 Park Center Court, Suite 300, Owings Mills, MD 21117
SH141A

Gramercy Books® and colophon are registered trademarks of
Random House Value Publishing, Inc.

Random House
New York • Toronto • London • Sydney • Auckland
http://www.randomhouse.com/

Printed and bound in the United States of America.

Library of Congress Cataloging-in-Publication Data
Chichester, Brian.
    Natural healing secrets : an a-to-z guide to the best home remedies /
Brian Chichester ; foreword by Dian Dincin Buchman.
        p. cm.
    1. Naturopathy—Popular works. I. Buchman, Dian Dincin.
II. Title.
RZ440.C465   1998
615.5´35—dc21

ISBN 0-517-16046-3   97-52138
                                                      CIP

8 7 6 5 4 3 2 1

DEDICATION

This book is dedicated to my truest source of health and happiness, my beloved parents and wonderful family. I would also like to thank the supporters of complementary medicine, and the researchers who ensure its safety and effectiveness.

NOTE TO THE READER

The information in *Natural Healing Secrets* is designed to help you increase your knowledge of home remedies that may relieve health problems in some cases. This book is intended as a reference resource only, and not as a substitute for proper and prompt medical care. Use this volume to complement, not to replace, any treatment or advice your physician may prescribe or recommend. For best results, seek your physician's approval before using any methods or remedies listed in this book.

TABLE OF CONTENTS

FOREWORD

Natural medicine has its origin in healing practices that have endured since the dawn of humankind. This observe-nature, pass-it-on-to-others style of medicine flowered eons before the unfolding of scientific medicine, and even today it continues to develop alongside modern medical research and practice.

Once primarily based on religion and magic, medicine gradually became more specialized. One example of this specialization is described in *The Healing Hand*, a masterful history of medicine by Dr. Guido Manjo. Manjo describes his puzzlement at finding that ancient Egyptian writings show that in 500 out of 700 or so medicinal remedies, honey is the main ingredient. To discover its purpose, Manjo conducted chemical experiments and discovered that honey breaks down chemically to a formula much like the modern antiseptic, hydrogen peroxide!

Modern medicine was first practiced by the Greek physician Hippocrates in the fourth century, but there have always been lay healers in villages throughout the world who cared for the sick with natural remedies. Many of the most enduring secrets found in this book come from the villages of Europe, from Native American settlements, and from ancient China.

In his book *American Indian Medicine*, Virgil Vogel reports that many of the plants discovered and used by Native Americans still appear in modern scientific medicine. Another ancient record of natural healing is *The Yellow Emperor's Nei Ching* or *Classic of Internal Medicine* The first written source of ancient Chinese medicine, the *Nei Ching* describes herbal cures, acupuncture, and many forms of meditation—concepts that have been used for many centuries and that now are incorporated in today's holistic medicine.

My own link to practical, natural medicine based on ancient remedies is deeply rooted in my family history. My maternal grandmother grew up in a remote European inn where her innkeeper father sometimes was called upon to heal local villagers. Surprisingly, my great-grandfather was accepted by and exchanged plant lore with local and passing Gypsies, who—then as well as today—did not readily embrace strangers. Because he befriended them, the Gypsies in turn taught their closely guarded healing secrets to my grandmother, whom they dubbed "Peaches and Cream." She passed on many of these healing secrets to me.

Closer to home, my dad, "Doc" Dincin, was a pharmacist who studied pharmacognosy, or the use of plants for medicine. He later used this profound knowledge as an advocate and practitioner of natural medicine. Among the things our family did every day was to eat a lot of fresh vegetables, and there were always huge salads at lunch and supper. I didn't realize that this "natural medicine" was considered bizarre until a cousin recently mentioned, "Can you believe it, Dian? My parents snickered at your parents because you ate *salads!*"

It is hard to believe today. But thus does life evolve. At last, the sensible old natural ideas are beginning to be understood and accepted. Simple and effective natural remedies, such as those my father inherited and learned, are of vital interest now.

I am passionately immersed in the science, history, and practicality of preventive medicine, so I was intrigued when the publishers of *Natural Healing Secrets* approached me to write a foreword to this book. The author of *Natural Healing Secrets* is a personal trainer and experienced health writer who truly understands the concept of a preventive medicine lifestyle. This book has much to offer the modern reader. Here you will find medical facts as well as easy, practical answers to a host of ordinary health problems. Neither Brian Chichester nor I advocate giving up one's alliance to a personal physician. But as he so aptly says in his introduction, in this day of managed care we have less time than ever with our doctors, and thus the deep bond that we once enjoyed with a family physician is now more fragile. Personal survival demands that we all learn more about preventive and natural approaches to life and living.

The object of this book is to *help you stay healthy*. It directs you to prudent lifestyle changes and the importance of careful eating and regular exercise. It provides healing secrets extracted from both historical sources and contemporary wisdom. The home remedies presented in *Natural Healing Secrets* are culled from those judged the safest and most prevalent.

Use them in good health!

Dian Dincin Buchman, Ph.D.

New York

Dian Dincin Buchman, who holds a doctorate in Health Sciences, is the author of: *Ancient Healing Secrets*, *Herbal Medicine*, *The ABC's of Natural Beauty*, *The Complete Herbal Guide to Natural Health and Beauty*, and *The Complete Book of Water Therapy*.

INTRODUCTION

You may remember a time when your family doctor was almost completely in charge of your health. He—family doctors were invariably men—seemed to know the secrets of life and death. He healed the sick and strengthened the weak. He trained in his art for almost a decade and was filled with wisdom. He knew what was good for you and your family. He gave wise counsel when you complained of stress and anxiety. He knew why your son broke out in hives when he ate spaghetti, and what your spouse should do about a tricky stomach.

Many of us still rely on a wonderful family doctor. But more and more, the face of health care is changing. No longer do we have just one doctor—we have specialists. Where you once spent twenty or thirty minutes with your doctor, now you're often rushed through a fifteen-minute exam after waiting an hour to be seen. The cost of each visit is skyrocketing, too, as is the cost of prescriptions.

The good news is that the United States has more than 500,000 practicing physicians and is among the most scientifically advanced, healthiest nations in the world. Thanks to a growing number of scientists entering the field, the advent of powerful technology, and expanded media coverage we know more about our health than ever before. And for the first time, we're becoming more proactive in maintaining it. We want to be involved in our health care. We're more sophisticated consumers. We're less likely to take our doctor's word as the only option, and we're more likely to seek a second or even a third opinion.

The comforts of home remedies. There's no need to wait until sickness strikes before you do something good for yourself. Nor do you always have to turn to doctors to treat aches and pains. There are ways you can treat many

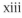

common health problems yourself—ways that don't require a lot of money, are effective, and can be done simply and safely at home. These home-remedy alternatives are the basis of natural healing, a concept that's been around for thousands of years.

But natural healing isn't for everyone—and certainly isn't appropriate for every condition. Some illnesses should never be self-treated. There clearly are times when you need to pursue the best medical attention you can find. Modern medicine and your family doctor can play a crucial role in maintaining your health, and it would be foolish to go without them entirely. (That's why most sections in this book include tips on when to see the doctor.) Natural healing supplements your physician's care. People who practice natural health care believe that many common problems—like a sinus attack, a headache, or indigestion—may benefit from a safe, proven remedy you can do yourself. In many cases, it doesn't hurt to try something at home before making an appointment to see your health practitioner.

Natural healing, as the name suggests, is based on the rich bounty of the earth and the healing wisdom of your own body. It's safe, effective self-help that's been around for ages.

Healing naturally. *Natural Healing Secrets* won't turn you into Hippocrates. It won't make your family doctor or other medical specialists obsolete. But it will guide you in keeping you and your family healthy. And you'll have plenty of company: One-third of all Americans have used so-called alternative or natural healing methods or home remedies for various conditions at some time in their lives.

Today, we are exposed to more helpful information and more healthful options than ever before. But with information comes misinformation. With their urgent deadlines, newspapers, magazines, and television can't always present the big picture.

What makes *Natural Healing Secrets* different is that we've taken our time. We've scoured the medical journals, the scientific studies, the book racks, the magazines, and the newspapers so you don't have to. We've sifted through thousands of home remedies, choosing only the very best. As a result, we've compiled the safest, most effective, and proven natural healing secrets you can find. What's more, most of these remedies work without any special ingredients or gadgets. You won't have to hack your way through a jungle for some rare, exotic plant to use our advice. Most of these remedies use what's already in your kitchen cabinet or what you can find at a health-food store, garden center, or over-the-counter at your pharmacy. In some cases, there are no ingredients at all—your tools are simply a firm touch of the hands or a change in what you eat or how you exercise.

Exploring the wonderful world of home remedies will be an exciting (and cost-saving) adventure for you and your family. Imagine taking care of common health nuisances, such as annoying hiccups or a painful earache, in the comfort of your own home. Imagine turning your window box or backyard into a medicine cabinet full of healing herbs. Imagine learning how to prevent many health problems in the future. With this book you'll realize all of these goals—and more. And it's easy to find just the remedy you need. Just look up whatever condition is bothering you—and you're on your way to natural good health!

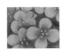

ACNE

We usually think of acne as a teenage problem—as though pimples and blackheads appear just in time for the prom, then disappear for the rest of your life. But acne can strike at any age. Doctors estimate that 5 percent of adults will have acne outbreaks at some time during their lives.

This is why: Your skin is packed with tiny oil-producing glands called sebaceous glands. Periodically these glands produce large amounts of oil, which can block the openings, or ducts, of the glands. When the oil can't get out, pressure builds. The walls of the ducts begin to swell, forming pimples.

The sebaceous glands are influenced by hormones, which is why acne often appears during the teenage years. But it can also be caused by hormonal fluctuations later in life—due to the menstrual cycle, for example, or to birth-control pills. People who are taking steroids for medical problems will also sometimes develop acne. Even the regular use of makeup or suntan oil, which can block pores, may cause an eruption.

You can't always prevent acne, but there are ways to keep those unsightly blemishes at bay. Here's how.

WHEN TO SEE THE DOCTOR

If your acne appears in cycles and you suspect it's related to hormone levels, or if the pimples are painful, infected, or persistent, you should see a dermatologist.

Keep your skin clean. Since acne is often caused by blocked pores, keeping your skin clean is one of the best ways to help prevent it. Wash your face once or twice a day with soap and warm water. Gentle washing is all that's required—pores easily unclog with a soft touch. Avoid using too much pressure or washing with harsh, abrasive cleansers, which will make the problem worse by irritating the skin.

Take direct action. For mild acne, over-the-counter products containing benzoyl peroxide can be very helpful. These topical products cause the skin to peel slightly, releasing trapped oils and bacteria and helping the inflammation heal.

Go easy on the makeup. Covering your skin with large amounts of makeup will clog pores, trap oils, and make it easier for pimples to form. To keep pores open, it's best to use makeup sparingly. It's also a good idea to use water-based makeups that are easily removed with gentle washing.

Let nature take its course. Even though pimples will go away on their own, it's easy to get impatient and give them a squeeze to hurry things along. But squeezing pimples can force the material in them deeper under your skin, leading to infection, inflammation, and possibly scarring. This is why doctors recommend you leave your skin alone.

Stay on top of stress. There's little scientific evidence that stress causes acne, yet most people notice that pimples do tend to flare up during stressful periods—before a wedding, for example, or when preparing for a job interview. You can't completely eliminate stress, but there are ways to keep it from leaving its mark on your skin. Getting regular exercise, meditating, or simply getting out to a movie now and then will help keep your whole body, including your skin, much healthier.

Eat well. Despite what you always hear, chocolate, French fries, and other high-fat foods don't cause acne.

But research suggests that foods high in iodine, such as fish, may contribute to acne outbreaks. The same is true of salty foods such as chips. It isn't necessary to revamp your entire diet when you're trying to control acne. But eating less "junk" may make a difference. It's also important to eat simple, healthy foods, like whole-grain breads, fruits, vegetables, and legumes. Foods that are high in fiber can help regulate hormone levels, which will help keep your complexion clear.

AGE SPOTS

Every carnival has an "age-guesser"—someone who will guess your age or you win the prize. They almost always win because they know one important secret: More than the face or hair, the skin on the hands can truly reveal a person's age.

Most people get age spots, also called "liver spots," at some time during their life. Age spots are flat patches of increased pigmentation, light brown or black in color, that range from the size of a freckle to several inches across. They occur most often on the backs of the hands and the arms, and sometimes on the face as well. Age spots are a harmless, but annoying sign of the march of years.

You can't prevent age spots entirely, but there are ways to make them less noticeable and also to prevent them in the future. Here are some tips you may want to try.

3

WHEN TO SEE THE DOCTOR

Although age spots are harmless, any new growth should be checked by a doctor to make sure it's not cancerous. If a spot or growth is bleeding, is changing color or size, or is itching or tingling, you should make an appointment right away. Skin cancer is serious, but it's usually easy to treat as long as you catch it early.

Lighten the spot. There are a number of over-the-counter products, called bleaching creams, that will help lighten age spots until they're barely noticeable. A less-expensive option is to make your own bleaching solution. Simply squeeze the juice from a lemon or lime—or use a blender to juice a red onion—and apply the juice from any of these to the spot with a cotton swab. Doing this twice a day for up to six weeks will substantially lighten or even eliminate small age spots.

Find a friend in vitamins. Some experts believe that getting more vitamins C and E in your diet is an excellent strategy for fighting age spots. These vitamins, which are known as "antioxidants," help neutralize harmful oxygen molecules that damage cells throughout the body, including in the skin. You can get plenty of vitamin C in foods such as citrus fruits, broccoli, and red and yellow peppers. It is also available in tasty chewable tablets. Vitamin E is a bit trickier to get because it's found mainly in wheat germ and cooking oils—foods that you wouldn't eat big quantities of. To get more vitamin E, doctors often recommend taking a multi-vitamin that contains this skin-protecting nutrient. Check the label to be sure.

4

What's good on the inside of your body may also be good on the outside. You can buy creams containing vitamins C and E at your pharmacy. Rubbed directly on the skin, they can be very helpful for erasing age spots.

Live in a shady world. Despite the name, "age spots" have less to do with aging than with sun exposure. Most doctors say that age spots are caused by a lifetime's exposure to the sun's ultraviolet rays, which break down collagen and cause permanent changes in the skin's natural pigmentation. Because your hands and face get the most sun, these are the places where age spots are most likely to form. Your best strategy is to avoid prolonged sun exposure, especially from 10 a.m. to 2 p.m., when the sun's rays are strongest. It's also important to wear a sunblock—preferably one with an SPF (sun-protection factor) of fifteen or higher whenever you're outdoors.

Wear protective makeup. The problem with sunblocks is that it's not always convenient to use them. But you can get the same protection by using makeup and moisturizers that contain sunscreen. To get the best results, doctors recommend applying moisturizing sunscreens right after your morning shower, when they'll help lock in moisture that gives your skin that healthy glow.

ANXIETY AND PANIC ATTACKS

Maybe you've invited forty guests for a pot-luck dinner and all of a sudden you're beginning to wonder what you've gotten into. Your internal dialogue may sound something like this: "What was I thinking? I can't handle

5

this big a crowd! Besides, no one's going to show up anyway. If they do, they'll probably leave early because they're bored. Boy, I hope I bought enough wine. Is the house really clean? I think I forgot to scrub under the toilet rim."

Sound familiar? Nearly everyone will experience periodic bouts of anxiety and panic. It's normal to feel frightened by life's stresses—an upcoming job interview, meeting your in-laws for the first time, or having a dinner party. But sometimes these emotions spiral out of control, causing your heart to pound and your mind to go blank. Panic makes you feel as though the worst is about to happen—and that there's nothing you can do to stop it.

There will always be times when you feel like you're in over your head. But doctors have found that it's not stress itself but how you react to stress that determines whether you'll experience a little anxiety or a full-blown panic attack. Here are a few ways to give yourself a moment's peace and put the brakes on panic and fear.

WHEN TO SEE THE DOCTOR

Anxiety and momentary panic are common and entirely normal. For some people, however, even small setbacks can result in full-blown fear—not just for a few minutes, but for hours, days, or even months. If you find that you regularly feel like you're out of control, and are experiencing a rapid heartbeat, fast breathing, sweating, stomach problems, or other symptoms of anxiety, you should call your doctor or a counselor right away.

Take a deep breath. It sounds like a cliché, but taking deep, regular breaths is one of the best ways to keep panic and anxiety under control. People breathe very rapidly when they're anxious—a symptom doctors call hyperventilation. The problem with this rapid breathing is that it actually reduces the amount of oxygen in your body, which

6

makes you feel nervous and out of control. Taking slow, deep breaths, on the other hand, floods your body with oxygen, making you feel calmer. In addition, taking a few minutes to breathe deeply is like counting to ten; it gives you time to think and put things in perspective, instead of merely reacting to emotions.

The next time you feel panic coming on, stop what you're doing and take a deep breath. Breathe in slowly while counting to five. Hold the breath for one second, then slowly breathe out. Continue doing this for a minute or two. The surge of oxygen will help you feel calmer and more in control—and better able to handle the stress that's bothering you.

Get a whiff of relaxation. Your nose is one of your most powerful weapons for countering anxiety and panic. Evidence suggests that certain scents can stimulate feelings of calm and relaxation. A whiff of lavender or sandalwood incense, for example, can help take the edge off stress. So can the smell of baby powder or even a scented candle. Or you can simply sprinkle some cinnamon into a pot of boiling water. It will fill the air with a delicate, lovely smell that reminds many people of simpler, calmer times.

"B" calm. The B vitamins are nature's stress relievers. Studies have shown that people who don't get enough B vitamins in their diets may experience confusion, anxiety, or irritation. You can get a lot of B vitamins by eating a healthful diet. But when stress and anxiety are riding high, you may want to take a B-complex multivitamin, which will help fortify your emotional defenses.

Take some herbal relief. For thousands of years, people around the world have been finding emotional strength in the garden. Herbs such as chamomile, ginkgo, kava, valerian, and St. John's Wort have been shown to help ease

7

panic and anxiety. In fact, recent studies suggest that St. John's Wort may be as effective as some prescription drugs for imparting feelings of calm and well-being. You can buy these healing herbs at natural food stores or from natural apothecaries. Many people prefer to buy dried herbs and make a tea, but the herbs are also effective when used in capsule form. When taking herbal supplements, however, be sure to read the label carefully to make sure you're taking the proper amount.

Put water to work. When your emotions are running high and you feel as though you're about to collapse, nothing is more soothing than taking a long, relaxing bath. Many people prefer their baths hot, but before you fill that tub full of steaming hot water, keep this in mind: Some experts believe that a lukewarm or slightly cool bath does a better job of relieving tension and anxiety. Fill the bath with water until it registers ninety degrees (you can pick up bath thermometers at most department stores) and soak for about twenty minutes, adding hot or cool water to keep the temperature constant.

Rub yourself the right way. Massage is one of the quickest ways to take the edge off panic and anxiety. There's a good reason for this. Massage improves the circulation, removes waste products like lactic acid from the muscles, and helps take your mind off stress and anxiety. And, it just plain feels good. Even if you don't feel like having a professional massage, it's easy to take ten to fifteen minutes a day to indulge yourself in a little self-massage. Take a few moments to rub your neck. Run your fingers across your scalp. Squeeze your shoulders, your thighs, and your calves. You can even try rolling a tennis ball along your arms to relieve tension, or roll a rolling pin on the long muscles of your upper legs. Doing this regularly will help lower stress and ease your anxiety.

Walk off your stress. Many people, when they first start feeling anxious, put on their sneakers and head outside. Taking a long walk—or, if you're athletically inclined, a jog or a bike ride—is one of the best ways to put the brakes on panic attacks. Research has shown that exercise can increase your tolerance to stress and make you more optimistic and upbeat. And it doesn't take a lot of exercise to get the benefits. Walking, swimming, or even dancing several times a week will help you feel more confident and in control—and less vulnerable to anxiety.

Experts usually recommend exercising three or four times a week for about half an hour each time. On days when you feel particularly anxious, you may want to exercise longer to work out your worries and frustrations.

Be careful what you eat. Just as some foods, like carbohydrates, can help you feel calm and relaxed, others can put your nerves on edge. When you're feeling stressed, it's a good idea to avoid drinks containing such things as caffeine and alcohol, which can boost your anxiety levels. During high-stress times, you may want to drink soothing, non-caffeinated herbal teas or simply some ice water flavored with lemon or lime. You should also avoid sweets and eat more filling "comfort" foods, such as potatoes, pasta, or whole-grain breads.

Turn off the internal chatter. Many doctors believe that negative thinking can have a profound impact on how we feel. Unfortunately, negative thoughts are hard to avoid. Remember that dinner party example at the beginning of this chapter? We all get panicky from time to time. But many of us have the equivalent of little tape machines in our heads that are constantly playing irrational and negative messages: "I'm losing control," or "I'm so stupid, what was I thinking?" Sound familiar? If so, you can turn things

9

around by changing what's on the tape. Start "playing" positive messages: "I'm strong. I'm in control. I'm nervous, but that's OK." If you constantly replace negative thoughts with positive ones, you'll find that they have a way of coming true. You'll still experience stress and anxiety, but you'll feel better able to handle them—and this is the key to keeping panic under control.

ARTHRITIS

Arthritis is an incredibly common condition, affecting about eight out of ten Americans at some time in their lives. While there are many types of arthritis, they all cause pain, stiffness, and swelling in the joints. People with arthritis may have trouble getting out of bed in the morning or bending over to tie their shoes. In some cases, the joints get so stiff and achy that even fastening a button can seem like an impossible task.

Even though there are more than one hundred kinds of arthritis, the two most common forms are osteoarthritis and rheumatoid arthritis. Osteoarthritis, also known as "wear and tear" arthritis, occurs when cartilage in the joints breaks down—as a result of injuries or too much weight, or simply a lifetime of repeated bending, flexing, and shifting. When the cartilage is damaged, bones begin rubbing against each other, causing pain. This can make even the most simple task, such as opening a jar, difficult to face.

Rheumatoid arthritis also causes cartilage to weaken and bones to rub. Unlike osteoarthritis, however, it's not simply caused by wear and tear. For reasons that aren't yet clear, rheumatoid arthritis causes the immune system to begin attacking the joints, wearing away cartilage and causing the joints to become inflamed and very tender.

Even though the different types of arthritis act in different ways, many of the remedies are the same. At present, arthritis can't be cured, but there are many things you can do to relieve pain and swelling and to help keep your joints mobile.

WHEN TO SEE THE DOCTOR

Doctors can be helpful in prescribing a program of treatment that suits you. Also, if you are considering a fast to lose weight, you should only do this under a doctor's care.

Relief as close as your kitchen. You wouldn't think that what you put on the menu would have any marked effect on arthritis, but research suggests that some foods, like asparagus, garlic, and onions, can help. These foods contain sulfur compounds, which can help your body repair damaged tissue throughout the body, including the tissue in the joints.

Get more vitamin C. This all-purpose nutrient has been shown to help relieve a variety of problems, including arthritis. Vitamin C is an antioxidant, which means it helps block the effects of harmful oxygen molecules in the body. It has also been shown to help the immune system work more efficiently. This can help ease inflammation in the joints and arthritis pain.

You can get plenty of vitamin C by eating a variety of fruits and vegetables, including citrus fruits, broccoli, and peppers. Many doctors also recommend taking a vitamin C supplement to maximize your intake.

11

Help from a special fat. Most of us are trying to cut back on the amount of fat we eat, but one type of fat, called gamma linolenic acid (GLA), can help fight swelling in the joints as well as calm the immune system in people with rheumatoid arthritis. You can find this fatty acid in oils, nuts, and fish. To get the most benefit, experts recommend eating cold-water fish, such as mackerel, tuna, salmon, sardines, and bluefish, at least twice a week.

You can also find this fatty acid in primrose oil, borage oil, and black currant oil, which are available in health food stores. When taking these or other fatty acid supplements, read the label carefully to make sure you're getting the proper amounts.

Consider cayenne. Cayenne contains a substance called capsaicin, which has been shown to block chemicals in the body that are responsible for transmitting pain signals to the brain. Of course, you'd have to eat a lot of cayenne pepper to get the benefits. An easier strategy is to take cayenne capsules, which are available in health food stores. Your doctor also may recommend using capsaicin cream, such as Zostrix, which is available in drugstores.

Put it on ice. One of the quickest ways to stop arthritis pain is to apply cold to your aching joints. You can use cold packs, or simply wrap ice cubes in a washcloth or towel and apply it for fifteen or twenty minutes, several times a day. A shortcut is to use a bag of frozen peas.

Or try some heat. Putting hot towels or a heating pad on painful joints will help increase blood flow, which can also relieve pain and ease swelling and stiffness.

12

Keep your weight in check. If you've wanted to lose weight, but haven't, here's another reason to try again. Carrying extra weight puts additional strain on your joints, increasing their wear and tear, and making them more likely to hurt when arthritis flares. In fact, there's some evidence that extra body fat increases arthritis even in joints that don't bear body weight.

Keep your joints moving. Regular exercise is a powerful ally in fighting arthritis pain as well as in preventing it in the first place. Exercise helps in several ways. It helps strengthen muscles surrounding the joints, so they provide more support. Keeping the joints moving also increases their internal lubrication so they move more easily and with less strain.

Taking walks once or twice a day is a superb exercise for people with arthritis. Not only will walking strengthen muscles, it is relatively low impact, so it puts very little stress on the joints. Swimming and bicycling are also good for easing and preventing arthritis pain.

When starting an exercise program, be sure to start out slowly. Doing too much all at once will only make your joints hurt more. As a rule, doctors recommend exercising three or four times a week, for twenty to thirty minutes each time. And don't forget to warm up by stretching for several minutes before putting your body in motion. This will help keep muscles and joints limber, so you don't hurt yourself along the way.

Make simple changes. When arthritis flares, even the simplest things—like raking the yard or opening a door—can be painful. There are many small changes you can make that will make life easier. For example, replace door knobs (which can be hard to turn) with easy-to-lift levers. Buy an electric can opener to replace your hand-held model. Some people even shop for clothes with zippers instead of buttons. Little changes, to be sure, but over time they can make your life a lot more comfortable.

ASTHMA

Nothing is more natural than breathing—unless you have asthma, in which case every breath can seem precious.

Doctors estimate that 10 percent of children and 5 percent of adults in America have asthma. Doctors still aren't sure what causes asthma, although the symptoms—coughing, wheezing, shortness of breath, and tightness in the chest—are all too familiar. Asthma causes tiny airways in the lungs to get swollen and inflamed. It also causes the body to produce more mucus, which makes breathing even harder.

One of the most frightening things about asthma is how suddenly it can appear. Exposure to pollen or other allergens, vigorous exercise, or even taking a breath of cold air can trigger an attack. So can a bout with the flu or even a common cold. Asthma attacks can last anywhere from a few minutes to several days. In severe cases, people need to go to the hospital because they simply can't breathe.

Asthma always needs to be under a physician's care. But there are many things you can do at home to make it a little better.

WHEN TO SEE THE DOCTOR

If you've started wheezing when you exercise, don't chalk it up to aging. It could be asthma, and you need to see your doctor right away. Without treatment, asthma can be life-threatening. With proper care, however, it can be controlled. A variety of medications, including steroids, are very effective at relieving symptoms and preventing future problems.

14

Brew some parsley tea. Parsley is a natural expectorant that can help clear mucus from the airways. When you are having an attack, sipping a cup of parsley tea will help you breathe more easily. To make the tea, steep a few sprigs of dried parsley in a cup of boiling water. As an additional benefit, steam from the tea will help loosen mucus and provide quick relief.

Pour a cup of coffee. Doctors often urge people to drink less coffee. But if you have asthma, a cup of joe may be just the thing. The caffeine in coffee is chemically related to a commonly used asthma drug. Having a cup or two of coffee when you feel an attack coming on will quickly cause airways to relax, making it easier to breathe.

Take a sweet Chinese remedy. We think of it as a sweet candy, but in Asian countries, people traditionally have used the herb form of licorice to help treat asthma. Some experts believe licorice has a mild anesthetizing effect that can ease the coughs that often accompany asthma attacks. You can buy licorice supplements in tablet form at health food stores. Licorice candy doesn't work, however, because it contains only trace amounts of the healthful elements. (If you have high blood pressure, don't take licorice, because it may make your condition worse.)

Clear the air. To keep your lungs in good working order, make sure everything you do is lung-friendly. For starters, don't allow people to smoke in the house. It's also helpful to cover your mattresses with dust covers to cut back on skin dander—tiny flakes of skin that can trigger allergies along with asthma attacks. Your doctor may also recommend that you buy a portable air filter that will help remove irritating particles from the air before they get into your lungs.

Unfortunately, doctors have found that there are more than 2,000 substances that can trigger asthma attacks— and that's only inside your house. Outside there may be thousands more. So you need to do everything you can to

15

keep the air you breathe clean. At the very least, it's a good idea to keep your windows closed and to use central air conditioning during the warm months. This will help trap airborne particles before they reach your lungs.

Read labels carefully. Some people with asthma find that aspirin, ibuprofen, and other over-the-counter pain medications can bring on severe attacks. In addition, foods containing sulfites, such as preserved meats, may trigger asthma attacks in some people.

Take care of your tummy. Doctors have found that heartburn may play a role in causing asthma attacks. Heartburn occurs when irritating stomach acids back up into the esophagus (the tube that connects the mouth to the stomach) and throat. The resulting irritation may trigger breathing problems. To prevent heartburn, it's best not to eat big meals late at night. Instead, eat smaller meals throughout the day, and eat a small dinner early in the evening. Some people also prop themselves up with pillows, which can help keep stomach acids where they belong. (For more on Heartburn, see page 85.)

Keep under wraps. Cold, dry air makes breathing difficult for everyone, especially people with asthma. In the winter, it is a good idea to wear a scarf around your nose and mouth when venturing outdoors. This will warm and humidify the incoming air, which will help keep your airways calm. In addition, you may want to use a humidifier indoors to moisten the air.

Pay attention to your hormonal cycles. Research suggests asthma might be influenced by the levels of various hormones in your body, particularly estrogen levels in women. Many women with asthma tend to have attacks just before or during the menstrual periods. If you notice that your breathing problems correspond with your monthly cycle, call a doctor.

He or she may recommend medications that will help keep your hormone levels more stable throughout the month.

Learn to relax. Several studies suggest that stress may play a role in bringing on asthma attacks. Doctors often recommend that people with asthma do their best to relax more often. This can be as simple as giving yourself time every day to do something you enjoy, or as intricate as taking up tai chi or meditation. It really doesn't matter what you do as long as it helps keep you calm and relaxed. Don't think of rest and relaxation as luxuries. For people with asthma, regular rest is as important as taking proper medications.

Start an asthma file. One of the worst things about asthma is that it's unpredictable. It can be hard to pinpoint what's most likely to cause an attack, and what will calm it down. To figure out your asthma "triggers," start keeping an asthma file. Whenever you have an attack, write down what you were doing when it occurred. Was it hot or cold outside? Were you active or sitting still? Excited or depressed? What did you have to eat that day? The more information you can accumulate, the easier it will be to figure out what's contributing to your problems—and what you need to do to stop them.

ATHLETE'S FOOT

We often think of athlete's foot as a condition suffered mainly by teenagers. After all, they're the ones tracking around in dirty locker rooms and wearing sneakers without socks. But don't kick your feet up and relax just yet. Anyone can get athlete's foot, and you don't have to walk around a locker room to catch it.

The term "athlete's foot" really isn't accurate because it has nothing to do with exercise or sports. Athlete's foot is caused by a mold-like fungus that thrives just about everywhere on your body—on your hair, skin, and around your nails. Most of the time it doesn't cause any problems. But occasionally the fungus is able to survive and thrive. When it does it can cause a variety of itchy skin infections—not only athlete's foot, but also such things as jock itch and ringworm. The athlete's foot fungus thrives in warm, damp places, which is why it grows so well on bathroom (or locker room) floors or on the insides of shoes.

WHEN TO SEE THE DOCTOR

Athlete's foot is rarely serious and will usually go away with home treatments. If the infection lasts more than a few weeks, however, you should see your doctor. There are other skin infections that resemble athlete's foot but persist without medical attention. You should also see your doctor if the itching gets worse or begins to spread.

18

It's impossible to avoid the fungus entirely, but there are ways to keep it under control and to prevent infections from taking hold. Here's what experts recommend for healthy, fungus-free feet.

Kill it with garlic. For ages, Russians have used garlic to relieve athlete's foot infections. There's some evidence they're on the right track. Garlic contains natural chemicals that kill a variety of organisms, including the athlete's foot fungus. The next time you have an infection, you may want to try peeling and mincing a clove of garlic, putting it in your sock, and wearing the sock to bed. Do this every night for a few nights. You should start to see improvement within a few days. Or you can simply peel a garlic clove and rub it on the sore areas on your feet twice a day.

Keep them high and dry. Because athlete's foot thrives in warm, moist environments, you can keep it under control simply by keeping your feet dry. One of the simplest strategies is also the most comfortable—going barefoot. This allows air to circulate around your feet and between the toes, which makes it harder for the fungus to survive. After showering, walk around barefoot as long as you can, then dry your feet thoroughly before putting on your socks and shoes.

Give them all-day protection. The same antiperspirant that keeps your underarms dry will work on your feet, as well. Applying an antiperspirant to your feet after bathing will help prevent sweating, making it harder for the fungus to thrive.

Powder your toes. Another way to keep your feet dry is to add some baking soda to the insides of your shoes, or lightly sprinkle some over your feet to absorb moisture. Don't use cornstarch, however, which can encourage other types of infections.

Dry your shoes. To prevent athlete's foot from setting up shop inside your shoes, doctors recommend giving your shoes a good drying between wears. You can use a blow dryer, set on low, to dry the insides of your shoes. Or

19

make it a point not to wear the same shoes two days in a row, which will allow them to dry on their own. Putting your shoes on a sunny window ledge will help them dry more quickly.

Wash your feet regularly. By washing your feet with soap and water, paying particular attention to the area between your toes, you will help wash away the athlete's foot fungus and help prevent infections from taking hold.

Don't wear shoes without socks. Clean, fresh socks absorb moisture and keep your feet dry. Shoes are meant to be worn with socks. Stick with socks made from natural fibers, like cotton or wool. Other fibers don't absorb moisture as well.

Don't bother with flip-flops. There's nothing wrong with wearing sandals or flip-flops, but don't count on them to prevent infections. The key to prevention is keeping your feet dry, which open shoes won't do.

See your pharmacist. A number of over-the-counter athlete's-foot medications are designed to help kill the fungus. Doctors usually recommend using medicated powders rather than sprays because they have the added attraction of absorbing moisture. Using antifungal creams can add moisture to your feet, possibly making the infection harder to treat.

BACK PAIN

Your back is incredibly versatile. As children, we twist and tumble, roll and romp, without thinking twice about the fragility of our spine and its surrounding muscles. As adults, we continue to take our backs for granted. We sit for hours at a time, which is extremely hard on the back. We also use our backs to lift everything from bricks to clinging children or pets, often from awkward positions. Eventually, of course, things start going wrong.

Back injuries take a staggering toll on society, accounting for many missed days of work and millions of dollars in lost productivity. Eighty percent of adults fall prey to back pain at least once, and many people get it again and again.

While some back problems are serious, the vast majority can be treated at home. Here's what you can do to get "back" in action.

WHEN TO SEE THE DOCTOR

Even though most back problems will go away on their own, some are quite serious and need a doctor's care. When you've taken a hard fall, for example, or if the pain isn't getting better within a week or two, you should call your doctor. If you're experiencing more than just back pain—if you're having shooting pains in one of your legs, for example—you should call your doctor immediately.

Take three days of R & R. Most back problems will go away if you give the injured muscles, ligaments, and tendons time to heal. Spend a few days in bed if you're having more than mild pain. But don't lie around longer than that unless your doctor says to. Constant bed rest weakens muscles, which can make the pain worse. Doctors usually recommend resting for a few days, then slowly returning to your regular routine. If it still hurts, go back to bed for a day or two. And be sure to take frequent rest breaks while you're healing.

Cool it. Several times a day, apply ice packs wrapped in towels to your painful areas for fifteen to twenty minutes at a time, and repeat this several times a day. Applying cold can help relieve the swelling that often accompanies back pain.

Then warm it up. When the worst pain has died down, usually in a few days, change your treatment from cold to hot. Use a heating lamp, a hot water bottle, or a heating pad wrapped in a towel. Apply heat for fifteen to twenty minutes several times a day. This will help improve circulation and allow the injury to heal more quickly.

Take over-the-counter relief. Aspirin, ibuprofen, and other anti-inflammatory, pain-killing medications can be very helpful for easing back pain. Acetaminophen can also help relieve pain. It doesn't work for inflammation, however, so it's not always as effective as aspirin or ibuprofen.

Have a rub-down. A gentle massage is a great strategy for easing back pain. Massage improves circulation, helps eliminate lactic acid and other chemical wastes from the muscles, and may help relieve muscle spasms.

Take away stress. Stress doesn't cause back pain, but it can make the pain worse by causing muscles throughout your body to contract and tighten. It's hard to feel relaxed when your back is killing you, but there are ways to feel a little less stressed. Begin by breathing deeply for fifteen or twenty minutes. Taking slow, deep breaths floods the body with oxygen, which will help you feel calmer and help the muscles relax. While you're lying around, plug in a good

22

movie. Anything you can do to distract yourself will help those tender muscles in your back to relax.

Give it time. Most back pain subsides within two weeks, and up to 90 percent of all cases get better within six weeks. No one enjoys feeling under the weather that long, but getting impatient won't make you get better any faster, and it may make your pain worse.

Train your back. One of the best ways to prevent pain in the future is to train your back to be ache-resistant. This means strengthening your back muscles and improving your overall flexibility. Doctors usually advise people with back pain to embark on a regular exercise program, including lifting weights, to tone the muscles so they're better able to support the spine. Make sure to consult a doctor before beginning, however.

Flex yourself healthy. Flexibility is crucial for preventing backaches. Keeping your back limber means you'll be able to do all the things you enjoy—like working in the garden, bowling, or dancing up a storm—without getting tied up in knots later. A trainer at a health club or a community center such as a YWCA can teach you simple stretches that you can do for just a few minutes a day. Or you may get more ambitious and take up an entire flexibility program, such as yoga or even modern dance.

Learn how to lift. Whether you're picking up your socks or hefting a fifty-pound sack, always lift by bending your knees and letting the muscles in your legs support the burden. Your leg muscles are larger and stronger than the muscles along your lower back, and they're better able to withstand the strain. Always make sure your footing is firm, and never jerk or lunge to lift something. Lifting slowly and carefully will still get the job done, with a lot less risk of injury.

Sleep with your back in mind. You won't do your back a lick of good if you pamper it by day, only to ambush it at night. Make sure your mattress is firm, not sagging and soft. Sleep on your side with your knees bent and a pillow between them. If you sleep on your back, put a small pillow under your knees. Avoid sleeping on your stomach.

Protect your feet. Good shoes act like shock absorbers, reducing jolts to your back when you're walking or running. Wear shoes that fit properly, are in good condition (not too worn), and are designed for walking. Try to resist fashion ads that insist you must wear high heels. These are the worst shoes you can wear for back health. Stick to well-cushioned low heels or flats.

Improve your standing in life. Perfect posture isn't just for armed service personnel or law enforcement officers. Perfect posture—or at least improved posture—is for anyone who wants to avoid the agony of a backache. In fact, many cases of backache stem from bad posture habits: Too much slouching or leaning too far back can weaken your back's natural supports. Here's what doctors recommend for picture-perfect posture:

Standing: Imagine a string is connected to the top of your skull and is pulling your body upright. Your head should be upright with your chin slightly tucked in, so that your ears are over your shoulders. Your shoulders should be held back and level, with your back straight. Your stomach and buttocks should be tucked in.

Sitting: Sit upright, avoiding the natural tendency to slouch. Whenever possible, sit in chairs that provide good lower-back support. Or you can add a little support by slipping a pillow or a rolled-up towel between your back and the back of the chair. Your upper body should be straight. Your thighs should be level, and your feet should be firmly on the floor.

BAD BREATH

It's not the kind of problem that will win you sympathy. You won't receive get-well cards or find bouquets of flowers on your desk. But you may come to work one day and find a package of breath mints on your desk—or notice that people are standing a little farther away than they used to.

Everyone has bad breath from time to time—because of the anchovies on your pizza, for example, or the extra chili you put on your lunch-time enchilada. But when you have bad breath all the time, there may be more at work than today's lunch.

WHEN TO SEE THE DOCTOR

When you're having bad breath all the time, no matter how often you brush your teeth, you need to see your dentist. There's a good chance you have a touch of gum disease that's causing the odors. In addition, you may want to see your doctor because bad breath may be caused by a variety of physical problems, including a sinus infection, heartburn, or even diabetes or lung disease.

Most of the time, of course, bad breath is merely temporary. Here are a few ways to make your breath fresh again.

Freshen up with fennel. If you've ever eaten at an Indian restaurant you've probably noticed a bowl of tiny seeds in a dish by the door. They're fennel seeds, and they're a traditional remedy for freshening the breath after eating. Fennel seeds have a delightful licorice flavor and an aroma that lingers, making them very effective for bad breath.

25

Have something sprightly. We don't usually think of apples as being breath fresheners, but their crisp texture and slightly sweet taste make them a perfect choice for cleaning your mouth after a hearty meal. Other foods that act as natural breath fresheners include parsley and oranges. Oranges are particularly good because they contain citric acid, which stimulates the salivary glands. The extra saliva will help "rinse" your mouth and keep your breath clean.

Rinse after eating. Perhaps the easiest way to keep your breath clean is simply to rinse your mouth with water after eating. This will wash away food particles, which can lead to bad breath later in the day. While you're at the fountain, be sure to swallow some of the water, as well. It will help dilute whatever is in your stomach, so strong odors will be less likely to drift upstream.

Take care of your teeth. Gum disease is a common cause of bad breath, and up to 70 percent of us have it. Most gum disease can be prevented with simple tooth care. When you don't brush your teeth regularly, a sticky, bacteria-laden film forms on the surfaces of the teeth. Over time this can damage the enamel on the teeth and also lead to gum infections.

Doctors recommend brushing your teeth at least twice a day and flossing daily. Don't forget to brush your tongue, too, because it's a natural haven for bacteria as well as small particles of food. In addition, you may want to rinse your mouth with a mouthwash containing zinc, which will help neutralize mouth odors.

Try the sizzle of baking soda. Before all those minty mouthwashes and toothpastes came along, people often brushed their teeth with a mixture of baking soda and hydrogen peroxide. Doctors have since found that regular brushing with this mixture changes acid levels in your mouth, making it less hospitable to odor-causing bacteria.

Watch what you eat. No matter how much they please your taste buds, you're courting bad breath when you eat strong-flavored or spicy foods. The worst offenders include garlic, onions, salami, tuna, coffee, and alcoholic beverages. When you're trying to protect your breath, you may want to avoid fatty foods, as well, because they can create a strong odor during digestion.

BREAST TENDERNESS

For many women, breast pain is as regular as clockwork—or at least as regular as their menstrual periods. Doctors aren't sure why it occurs, but a woman's shifting levels of estrogen, progesterone, and prolactin may be accompanied by painful changes in the breasts. The breasts often retain fluids, causing them to swell. During the menstrual cycle the breasts add new cells to the milk-producing ducts and glands, which also makes them swell and get tender.

Since breast pain often occurs so regularly for so many years, many women simply resign themselves to feeling uncomfortable every month. But you don't have to put up with tender breasts. Here are some easy, effective strategies for keeping the discomfort under control.

Wear the right bra. The most effective way to control monthly breast pain is to wear a comfortable bra that provides good support. Doctors usually recommend that women wear a support bra rather than an underwire bra when their breasts are most tender. You may even want to wear the bra while you sleep. The bra should cup the breasts firmly, without binding or biting.

Try some cold comfort. You can take the same approach to tender breasts that you would for a sore back or a pulled shoulder muscle. Fill a plastic bag with ice cubes and wrap a towel around it. Then apply it to your tender areas for ten to fifteen minutes at a time. (You can also use commercial cold packs or the re-freezable packs that come with coolers.) This will slow the flow of fluids to the breasts, which will help reduce the swelling.

Add more fiber to your diet. Research has shown that eating foods high in dietary fiber, like fruits, vegetables, whole grains, and legumes, can help lower the amount of estrogen circulating in the bloodstream. For many women, this can help control monthly breast pain.

Cut back on salt. When you get a lot of salt in your diet the body begins retaining fluids, causing the breasts to swell. Eating less salt when your period is approaching will help reduce swelling as well as tenderness.

Trim fat from your diet. A diet that's high in fact isn't only bad for your heart—it can increase breast pain, as well. Experts believe that eating large amounts of fat can interfere with the production of chemicals in the body that are responsible for reducing breast pain. In addition, dietary fat has a way of turning into body fat, and fatty tissue has been shown to interfere with the body's ability to regulate estrogen. Doctors recommend getting no more than 20 to 25 percent of your total daily calories from fat. The best way to reduce fat in your diet is to cut back on the worst offenders—high-fat foods such as butter, red meats, margarine, mayonnaise, ice cream, and cheeses.

Cut back on coffee. American's favorite eye-opener may not be doing your breasts any good. There's little scientific

28

evidence that drinking coffee increases monthly breast pain, but many women have found that when they cut back on caffeine, the pain gets better.

Sip some herbal tea. As a substitute for coffee, you may want to try some uva ursi tea. Available in health food stores, this tea is a mild diuretic that can help ease breast pain by removing excess fluids from the body.

Try to stay active. Regular exercise has been shown to reduce the amount of fluids in the body, which can be very helpful for easing breast pain. You don't have to join a soccer team or run a marathon to get the benefits. Walking or riding a bike for twenty or thirty minutes three times a week, especially in the week before your period, can make a big difference in preventing (and relieving) breast pain.

WHEN TO SEE THE DOCTOR

Most monthly breast pain begins a few days to a week before menstruation, then goes away when the period starts. If the pain lasts longer, however, you should call your doctor. This is especially true if your breasts feel hot or lumpy, or if they're red or blotchy. You should also see a doctor if there's a discharge from the nipples, whether or not it occurs around the time of your period.

BRITTLE NAILS

Every day your fingernails put in hard labor—tapping on desktops, opening envelopes, digging in the garden, or scratching off the peel on instant-win lottery cards. Fingernails are incredibly strong and can usually withstand all the abuse we give them. After about age thirty, however, people's nails get weaker and more brittle. This can cause them to break or splinter, or simply look a little more ragged than they used to.

You can't prevent brittle nails entirely, but there are ways to make them a little stronger. Here's how.

Put some vegetables and beans on your plate. Lentils and peanuts, along with cauliflower, are rich sources of biotin, a B vitamin that has been shown to strengthen and thicken nails. But you need quite a bit of biotin—more than you can get from foods alone—to get the benefits. So when you're eating for nail strength, you may also want to supplement your diet with a multivitamin.

Add some fish to the menu. Salmon, mackerel, and other cold-water fish contain fatty acids, which the body uses to strengthen the nails. Eating fish several times a week will help keep your nails worry-free.

Keep them moist. Your fingernails naturally get hard and brittle whenever they dry out. To keep them moist, doctors recommend rubbing moisturizer around the nails once or twice a day. A little bit of petroleum jelly will also help keep the nails flexible and strong.

Don't let them soak. Your fingernails can absorb tremendous amounts of water. This sounds like it would be helpful for brittle nails, but it's actually just the reverse. Your nails expand when they absorb water, then contract when they dry. The more this cycle is repeated, the weaker the nails get. So it's worth keeping them dry whenever you can.

Enjoy a little elegance. Even if you don't go for rainbow colors, it's worth applying a little nail polish to strengthen nails and help them retain their natural moisture.

Avoid harsh chemicals. The problem with using fingernail polish is that you'll also be using fingernail polish remover, which usually contains acetone. Acetone quickly removes moisture from the nails. Whenever possible, use fingernail polish removers that do not contain acetone, doctors advise.

Treat them with respect. Fingernails are tough, but you didn't purchase them in a hardware store, so you shouldn't expect them to do double-duty as tools. Scissors, screwdrivers, staple removers, and tweezers were all invented for a reason. Use them, and give your fingernails a break. The less you use (and abuse) your nails, the stronger they are likely to be.

Cover them up. One of the best ways to protect brittle nails is to wear gloves whenever you're putting your hands to work in rough environments—in a sink full of hot, soapy water, for example, or in a mound of garden soil.

Keep them trimmed. Long nails are more fragile and break more easily than short ones. This is one reason to keep your nails short. To make the job easier, soak your hands in water for a few minutes first. Or trim your nails right after you've had a relaxing shower or bath.

31

BURNS

If you've ever brushed your arm against a hot oven rack or spattered your hands with hot drops of cooking oil, you know how painful even small burns can be.

Fortunately, the most common kind of burn, called a first-degree burn, isn't too serious. This is the sort of burn you get when you accidentally touch a hot iron or the handle on a cast-iron skillet. The surface of the skin gets red and sore, and there may be a little bit of swelling. Unlike the more serious second- and third-degree burns, most simple burns can be treated at home.

WHEN TO SEE THE DOCTOR

When you have a second- or third-degree burn, it's essential to see your doctor right away. You have a second-degree burn when the skin is oozing and blistering. Third-degree burns will leave the skin charred, turning it white or gray. Both types of burns can easily get infected and are potentially very serious. Even if you have what seems like a mild burn, you should call your doctor if it seems unusually painful or if it covers an area larger than two or three inches in diameter.

Get the water flowing. Make that a lot of water. When you've burned yourself, the heat quickly passes into the skin, possibly damaging tissues deeper inside. To cool the heat on the skin as well as below the surface, flood the area with cool, running water for at least fifteen minutes. Any less and the cool temperatures won't get to where the problem is. If you don't have access to running water—or if the burn is in an area that's hard to get to—you can apply a cloth that's been soaked in cold water. Ice wrapped

32

in a towel is also very helpful. (Don't apply ice directly to a burn because it can cause further skin damage.)

Once the burn is cool, gently pat your skin dry and apply an antibiotic ointment. In most cases, this is all you'll need to do to prevent blisters or swelling later on.

Spread on the aloe. People have been using the juice from aloe vera plants for centuries—not only for burns, but for relief from all kinds of skin injuries. Aloe vera contains a compound called allantoin, a substance that has been shown to speed wound healing. Better yet, it's a lot cheaper than over-the-counter drugs. Many people keep a plant on their windowsill—just in case!

Before using aloe vera, clean the burn thoroughly with soap and water. Then break off a piece from a leaf of the plant and cut it lengthwise. (You don't have to pick off the leaf—it will "heal" its own cuts and can be used again another time.) Squeeze out the gel and apply it liberally to the burn several times a day.

Try a milk compress. If you don't have aloe, you can also treat a burn with a milk compress. Like water, cool milk will quickly put out a burn's fire. In addition, the fat in milk may help burns heal more quickly. Leave the compress in place for five to ten minutes. Then rinse your skin well and pat the area dry.

Get some vitamin C. Your body uses this powerhouse nutrient to help repair damaged tissues, including those damaged by burns. For extra help in healing wounds, doctors often recommend getting 500 to 1,000 milligrams of vitamin C a day.

Put on some infection protection. Because even small burns can expose large areas of sensitive skin, there's a high risk of infection. To protect yourself, it's a good idea to apply an antibiotic burn cream, which will add moisture to

33

the wound and also prevent infections from taking hold. As an added benefit, antibiotic creams seal off the burn from the air, which can irritate exposed nerve endings.

Put aspirin to work. This all-purpose remedy is very effective at stopping the pain from burns. In addition, aspirin (as well as ibuprofen) can help stop inflammation, which will relieve pain and may help the area heal faster.

Let the burn breathe. It's a good idea to bandage burns, but you don't want to wrap the area so tightly that no air gets in. Doctors recommend dressing burns with sterile pieces of gauze. Don't wrap the gauze tightly in place, since this will only irritate the burn. Instead, wrap it lightly, which will protect it while allowing air to circulate.

Ban the butter. For years, people "treated" burns by smearing on butter or grease. Doctors now know that this old-fashioned practice actually makes burns worse because it locks in heat rather than allowing it to escape. Plus, putting butter or grease on a burn can promote infection.

BURSITIS AND TENDINITIS

Maybe you're starting to have trouble reaching high shelves. Or perhaps your tennis serve is getting a little stiff, or your elbows are feeling sore and creaky. When you can't move as easily as you used to, there's a good chance you have bursitis or tendinitis—conditions that can make your joints feel as stiff and rusty as the Tin Woodsman in the rain.

Bursitis occurs when one or more bursae—small, fluid-filled sacs that cushion the joints—get irritated and inflamed. Tendinitis also causes joint pain. Unlike bursitis, however, the irritation and inflammation caused by tendinitis affect the tendons, those sinewy fibers that connect muscles to bones.

Even though bursitis and tendinitis are different problems, it really doesn't matter which you have, because the treatments for both are virtually the same.

Do some quick first aid. When your joints first start aching, taking quick action will help prevent pain and swelling and speed your recovery time. Doctors recommend following a four-point plan called RICE: It stands for Rest, Ice, Compression, and Elevation, and it's the best way to quickly ease tendinitis and bursitis.

Resting your joints is the best way to help them recover. This is not the time to ignore the pain. Staying active when you're having tendinitis or bursitis will make the joints get worse in a hurry. Try to avoid the repetitive motion behind your condition for awhile, especially.

Once you're off your feet, it's time to start the next step of the program: Ice. When you first start having pain, put ice packs (or ice cubes wrapped in a towel) on the painful areas for fifteen to twenty minutes at a time. This will slow blood flow, which will help prevent swelling. After applying cold, wrap the painful area with an Ace bandage. Using compression will also help stop swelling, as well as reduce additional stress to the area.

Finally, you want to elevate the joint. If your shoulder is hurt, for example, sit up in bed for awhile. If it's your knee, prop your leg up with pillows. Elevating the area makes it harder for fluids to flow into the injured joint, which will reduce swelling and help ease the pain.

With the RICE approach, you can expect bursitis to start getting better within a week or two. Tendinitis is a bit more tenacious, however, and it may be a month or more before you're feeling entirely strong again.

Keep moving. Even though you don't want to put a lot of stress on already-sore joints, it's a good idea to stay somewhat active even when your joints are aching. Keeping the joints and muscles moving will help them stay loose and limber. In addition, moving actually helps lubricate the joints, so they move more easily. Doctors usually recommend taking several days to a week of complete rest—to give your "tennis" elbow a break, for example, or leaving your running shoes in the trunk of your car—until the worst of the pain is over. Then slowly begin resuming your normal activities, being careful not to push yourself too hard. Gradually moving your joints through their full range of motion will help speed healing as well as prevent problems in the future.

Try some soothing heat. After the initial pain has gone away and you're starting to feel a little better, you may want to put some heat—hot, moist towels, heat packs, or simply a heating pad—on the sore joints. The heat will improve circulation and can be very soothing for aching joints. As with cold, apply heat for about twenty minutes at a time. You can repeat this every few hours, or as often as is necessary to relieve the pain.

Block the inflammation. A lot of the pain caused by bursitis and tendinitis is due to inflammation. To stop swelling fast, doctors usually recommend taking aspirin or ibuprofen. These over-the-counter medications block the effects of chemicals in the body called prostaglandins that cause both pain and inflammation.

WHEN TO SEE THE DOCTOR

Although bursitis and tendinitis can be very painful, they'll usually clear up on their own. If the pain doesn't get better within a few weeks, however, you should call your doctor, who may recommend using powerful anti-inflammatory drugs such as steroids to stop the swelling, or some physical therapy you can try at home. For very severe cases of bursitis, you may need surgery to remove the troublesome bursa.

There's one other danger sign to watch out for. If you're having joint pain and the area is warm, red, and tender, you should call your doctor immediately. You could have a condition called septic bursitis, in which an infected joint spreads infection throughout your body.

CARPAL TUNNEL SYNDROME

It's only in the last few years that we've begun hearing a lot about carpal tunnel syndrome, a potentially serious condition in which the hands and wrists get tingly, numb, or sore. It's not a new condition, exactly, but the things that cause it—long hours spent doing repetitive tasks, like typing on a keyboard or working a cash register—have become increasingly common in our ever more high-tech, hands-on world.

Carpal tunnel syndrome gets its name from a channel in the wrist called (what else?) the carpal tunnel. When you use your hands and wrists a lot, tissues lining the carpal tunnel may get inflamed and swollen. If they start to press on a nerve in the wrist, you may have pain, numbness, or other symptoms.

37

Experts estimate that as many as half a million Americans have carpal tunnel syndrome. In fact, nearly half of all job-related injuries are caused by repetitive motions. People who do the same motions over and over again, like computer programmers, butchers, cashiers, and professional musicians—are those who have the highest risk of getting this painful condition. It can be serious because, once you get it, without proper treatment it may last a long time and prevent you from doing the things your job or daily life requires.

It would be nice if we could all give our wrists a rest from time to time, but that isn't always possible. Fortunately, there are other ways both to prevent and treat the pain of carpal tunnel syndrome. Here's what experts advise.

WHEN TO SEE THE DOCTOR

Because carpal tunnel syndrome involves the nerves, you should see a doctor at the first sign of problems. If you suspect you have it, here's a simple test: Hold the backs of your hands together in front of your body, with the fingers pointing down. Hold this position for about a minute. If your wrists begin to ache or you experience shooting pains in your hands or fingers, you should call your doctor right away.

Take a mini-break. Since carpal tunnel syndrome is caused by repetitive motions, it makes sense that giving your wrists a break from work will help prevent problems. Studies have shown, in fact, that simply taking "mini-breaks" from your usual job—by taking a few minutes to make phone calls, for example, or simply stretching your hands and wrists and wiggling your fingers—can relieve pain and protect the wrists from long-term harm.

Give your hands a shake. Many people with carpal tunnel syndrome have found that giving their hands and arms a quick shake will provide quick and effective temporary pain relief. Even dangling your arms for a few minutes can relieve painful pressure on the nerve.

Seek diversity. Just as taking a vacation can make you feel refreshed and relaxed, giving your hands a break from their usual tasks can have a similar effect. If you work a cash register all day, for example, you may not want to play the piano every night. Instead, look for activities that don't put additional stress on your hands and wrists—like taking walks in the evening or going dancing a few nights a week.

Consider a splint. The hands and wrists simply weren't designed for the constant pounding many of us give them every day. To provide additional support and protection, doctors often advise people with carpal tunnel pain to wear special splints that help stabilize the wrists and provide relief from pain. The splints, which are available in pharmacies, come on and off as easily as putting on a glove, and you can use them as often—or as rarely—as you feel is necessary. Some people don the splints only for tough jobs—when they're typing a long report, for example—and take them off as soon as they're done.

Get a grip. Whether your hobby is cooking, carpentry, or working in the garden, having tools with the proper handles can dramatically reduce the strain on your wrists. Simply placing foam rubber over the handles of brooms or hammers can make them much easier to grip. You can even buy can openers and kitchen knives that have thicker handles, which will make tasks like opening cans, slicing, dicing, and chopping a lot more comfortable.

Try hot and cold. Many people with carpal tunnel pain get quick relief by putting ice in a washcloth and holding it on their wrists for fifteen or twenty minutes. Conversely,

39

putting a heating pad on your wrist can quickly relax the muscles and help ease the pain.

Check your weight. Researchers aren't sure why, but people who are overweight appear to have a higher risk of developing carpal tunnel syndrome—possibly because fatty tissue can put additional strain on nerves and tendons in the wrists. Losing even small amounts of weight can help "open up" the carpal tunnel, reducing pain and helping prevent future problems.

Take some over-the-counter relief. When wrist pain is flaring, one of the best things you can do is take a few aspirin or ibuprofen. Often, these medications will quickly relieve pain as well as swelling.

COLDS

There's a good reason it's called the "common cold." Adults get colds an average of two times a year, and children usually come down with them a lot more often. Yet in some ways, the common cold is unique. Experts have identified more than 200 viruses that can cause colds, and the viruses are changing all the time. Even when your immune system learns to recognize one virus, there's always a different strain waiting to take its place.

40

Doctors have been trying for years—without success—to find a cure for the common cold. In the meantime, there's a lot you can do to reduce the symptoms and help your body get well.

WHEN TO SEE THE DOCTOR

Colds by themselves are rarely serious and will go away on their own. When you've been sick, however, the immune system may have a hard time protecting you against other infections. That's why people with colds will sometimes develop other, more serious conditions, like bronchitis or pneumonia. If your cold is lasting much longer than usual, or if your phlegm is thick and discolored, you may have picked up a "secondary" infection and you should call your doctor.

Take some echinacea. Echinacea is an herb that's renowned for its ability to strengthen the immune system. In fact, doctors in Europe recommend echinacea as much or more than some prescription drugs. You can buy echinacea in capsule, liquid, or even tea form at health food stores. Follow the directions on the label and take it as needed. Make sure you take it at the onset of a cold, however; it's much more effective in preventing colds that are "on their way in" than colds "on their way out."

Put vitamin C to work. This powerful vitamin has been shown to help neutralize the effects of harmful oxygen molecules in the body that can weaken the immune system. Studies suggest that getting lots of vitamin C can help relieve cold symptoms and even shorten the length of time that colds stick around.

You can get a lot of vitamin C in your diet, but when you're sick you may want to take a supplement. For colds, experts recommend taking 500 milligrams (or more) of vitamin C a day.

A chicken in every pot. For years, people have sworn that chicken soup helps relieve congestion and other cold symptoms. Modern research suggests it really can make a difference—and what a wonderful, comforting home remedy it is! When you feel the sniffles coming on, make a big

41

pot of chicken soup and enjoy it all day long. (Canned soup may help, but studies suggest that the home-made kind probably works better.) As an added benefit, sipping the hot liquid will help loosen congestion in your nose and throat, which will help you breathe more easily.

Some like it hot. Research has shown that eating spicy foods, like chili, hot peppers, or cayenne, can help break up congestion so you can breathe more easily. Even if you aren't in the mood for Mexican, Indian, or other spicy cuisines, you can get quick nose relief by mixing about a quarter-teaspoon of hot pepper powder in a glass of water and drinking it down. You can also buy cayenne capsules in health food stores.

Keep the fluids flowing. To ease the scratchy throat and dry eyes that often accompany colds, it's a good idea to drink plenty of water—at least eight to twelve glasses a day. Getting more fluids—not only water, but also fruit or vegetable juices—will help thin mucus in your nose and chest, so you'll feel more comfortable.

Keep your hands clean. The viruses that cause colds can live on the hands for a long time. Washing your hands several times a day is one of the best ways to prevent colds. Even if you're already sick, washing your hands will help prevent cold viruses from re-infecting you and prolonging the misery.

Take a long shower. A long, steamy bath or shower can work wonders for sore, crampy muscles that often accompany colds. And, the steam will help thin and loosen secretions in your airways, so you can breathe more easily.

Think about zinc. Research has shown that zinc lozenges can help sore throats heal more quickly and reduce the amount of time that you're sick—in some cases, by as much as several days, doctors say. Ask your local pharmacist about where you can obtain these pain-tamers.

COLITIS

The symptoms are uncomfortable and more than a little scary: abdominal pain, blood or mucus in the stool, diarrhea, cramping, urgent bowel movements, weight loss, and more. When you have colitis, a serious inflammation of the colon, you may feel as though you'll never be comfortable again.

Doctors aren't sure what causes colitis, although they think it may stem from infection or problems with the immune system. There also appears to be a genetic link—if your parents have colitis, you're at a higher risk of getting it, too. One of the worst things about colitis is that it's so unpredictable. In some cases it goes away for weeks, months, or even years at a time, then comes roaring back.

WHEN TO SEE THE DOCTOR

There isn't a cure for colitis, and it's not a problem you can treat at home. People with colitis or who suspect they might have it should always be under a doctor's care, and in many cases will need drugs or surgery to keep it under control.

There are things you can do at home, however, to reduce the symptoms and make this painful condition a little bit easier to live with.

Keep eating well. It's hard to keep up your appetite when your insides are acting up, but it's critical for people with colitis to eat plenty of vegetables, whole grains, and other nutritious foods. This condition can cause the body to lose enormous amounts of nutrients. Eating well as often as you can will help keep your body strong and able to cope.

43

But keep track of what you eat. For many people, certain foods appear to trigger colitis flare-ups, or to make the symptoms they're already suffering worse. There isn't one food that's right—or wrong—for everyone, so it's up to you to discover if certain foods are causing your problems. Doctors often recommend that people with colitis keep a food diary, in which they write down everything they're eating. That way, when your symptoms return, you'll be able to look back and see what may have contributed to the problem—and what you'll want to avoid next time.

Use fiber wisely. Research suggests that eating fruits, vegetables, and other fiber-rich foods can help prevent colitis flare-ups. On the other hand, eating fiber when you're already having symptoms may make you feel worse instead of better. Doctors usually recommend that people with colitis get plenty of fiber in their diets when they're feeling well, then cut back on it during bad times. During flare-ups, many people still eat fruits and vegetables, but peel them to remove a lot of the fiber. This is one time when you may want to use those canned goods you've been stockpiling in your cupboard—canned fruits and vegetables have less fiber than fresh.

Go easy on dairy. Many people with colitis have difficulty digesting lactose, a sugar in milk and other dairy foods. You may find that giving up dairy—or at least eating less of it—will help relieve your symptoms.

CONSTIPATION

We spend a lot of our lives waiting around. We wait in line at the grocery store. We wait for appointments that are two hours late. We wait for the kids to get home with the car. Who wants to have to wait for a simple bowel movement? It's no fun.

Unfortunately, this is one area where a lot of us—about 50 million Americans—do a lot of waiting. Constipation is extremely common, and for some people it happens all the time. Everyone's "schedule" differs, however. You may be on a normal timetable.

Although constipation is a simple problem, defining it gets a little more complicated. Doctors agree that there's no such thing as a "normal" bowel movement schedule. Some people have bowel movements twice a day, others three or four times a week. Just because you don't have a bowel movement every morning doesn't mean that you're constipated. As a general rule, doctors say that you're constipated if you don't have a bowel movement three times a week, or if you have other symptoms, as well, such as cramps or a lot of gas.

Many people turn to laxatives to have regular bowel movements. But most of the time these medications simply aren't necessary and can even be dangerous. A better choice is to make some simple changes in your diet and lifestyle. In most cases, just eating a little more fiber and getting more exercise and fluids is all you need to stop constipation for good. Here's what doctors advise.

45

WHEN TO SEE THE DOCTOR

Constipation is rarely serious, but when it lasts a long time or you're feeling very uncomfortable, you should call your doctor. This is especially true if there's blood in the stool or if you're having alternating bouts of constipation and diarrhea, which could be signs of more serious intestinal problems.

Begin with fiber. The most effective way by far to stop constipation—for good—is to eat more foods that are high in dietary fiber. Fiber is not digested as it moves through the intestines, and that's exactly why it's so helpful. Similar to a sponge, fiber absorbs tremendous amounts of water. When it reaches the colon it makes stools that much larger and easier to pass.

Doctors recommend getting twenty-five to thirty-five grams of dietary fiber a day. (The average American gets less than fifteen grams a day.) That sounds like a lot, and it would be if you ate it all at once. But if you eat more fruits, vegetables, whole grains, and legumes—not all at one meal, but throughout the day—you naturally get all the fiber you need, and then some. Even adding two or three fiber-rich foods to your diet every day—having oat bran for breakfast, for example, and a few slices of whole-grain bread at lunch, and a serving of vegetables and beans at dinner—may be all it takes to stop constipation for good.

H_2O—and hold the "joe." A lot of people simply don't drink a lot, and this can cause the stools to get dry and hard. Drinking eight to twelve glasses of water or juice a day will lubricate the insides of your intestines so stools move along more easily. Doctors often recommend that people drink two glasses of cold water every morning. Not only will you benefit from the extra fluids, but the cold water can "wake up" the intestines and start them moving. In fact, drinking more fluids is good for your general health.

Incidentally, coffee, colas, and caffeinated teas may be wet, but they aren't as effective as other fluids. In fact, they have a mild diuretic effect, meaning they can actually remove more fluids from your body than they add. Also, tea contains compounds called tannins, which may play a role in causing constipation.

Try a little rhubarb. Fresh rhubarb contains a lot of fiber, and it is a traditional remedy for constipation. Some experts recommend putting a little rhubarb in the blender and making a juice. Take a small amount at first, because for some people it can be very powerful and fast-acting. Only use rhubarb stalks, however, because the leaves can be toxic.

Put your hands to work. According to experts in acupressure, rubbing the fleshy area between your thumb and index finger can help stimulate many bodily functions, including digestion. Periodically pinching and rubbing this area, using light pressure, may help get your bowels moving again.

Stay active. When you move your body, your intestines will often get moving, too. Doctors have found that regular exercise can be essential for stopping constipation. Simply walking a few times a day, riding a bike, or even going dancing will keep all your muscles, including those in the digestive tract, working well.

CORNS AND CALLUSES

We take our feet for granted, but they're astonishingly complex. Each foot contains 26 bones, 100 ligaments, and 33 muscles, which work together in perfect harmony every time you take a single step.

But for all their complexity, our feet really weren't designed for the modern world. They spend their days and nights tightly encased in tennis shoes, sandals, or shiny black pumps. The constant friction causes skin on the feet to get thick and rough. In areas where they're constantly being rubbed the wrong way, the skin can form tough bumps called corns and calluses. They're really the same thing, although calluses are spread over a large area, while corns are quite a bit smaller.

Corns and calluses aren't a serious health threat, but they can make your feet feel tired and sore. They're also easy to get rid of. Here's what you need to do.

WHEN TO SEE THE DOCTOR

Corns and calluses rarely cause serious problems, but if your feet are extremely sore or are getting numb, you need to call your doctor. In addition, if you have diabetes or have poor circulation in your feet, don't try to treat corns or calluses yourself. Ask your doctor for advice.

Rub them away. Because corns and calluses are nothing more than thickened layers of skin, you can "erase" them by giving them a regular rub-down. After taking a bath or soaking your feet to soften the skin, gently rub the rough areas for a minute or two with a pumice stone or a foot file. Don't try to get rid of the whole thing all at once. Just gently remove the upper layers of skin. If you do this every day for a few weeks, the corns and calluses will gradually disappear.

Wear them away with aspirin. Another way to remove hard calluses is to crush several aspirin, then add a little lemon juice and water to make a paste. Apply the paste to the rough spots, then cover your foot with a warm towel and wrap the whole thing in a plastic bag. After about ten minutes, remove the wrappings and gently rub the callus with the pumice stone. This treatment is very safe and effective. Don't do it, however, if you're allergic to aspirin.

Pad the problem areas. When corns and calluses are hurting, you can get fast relief by padding the sore spots with a little bit of moleskin padding, which is available in drugstores.

Save the stilettos for special occasions. You may love the look, but high heels won't treat you well. Because of the design, high heels put a tremendous amount of pressure on the heels and the front of the feet. In fact, they're one of the leading causes of foot problems, including corns and calluses. There's nothing wrong with wearing high heels occasionally, but day-to-day you're better off wearing flats with larger, rounded toes and comfortably padded soles.

Try a change of socks. If your socks don't fit right they can rub against the skin with every step you take. Make sure your socks fit snugly and are thick enough to provide adequate cushioning. Once your socks begin to wear out, toss them out. Your feet will thank you for it.

Shop late in the day. Due to gravity, your feet naturally get larger as the day progresses. That's why a pair of shoes can feel just right in the morning, but be painfully tight later on. Doctors recommend buying shoes in the afternoon, when your feet are at their maximum size. This way, you won't buy shoes that are too small, which would make your feet susceptible to rubbing.

49

CUTS AND SCRAPES

It's hard to image a better covering than your skin. It keeps you warm, holds your insides in, and keeps the outdoors out. It's remarkably tough, and it even repairs itself when it gets worn or damaged. Just try to find another coat that does that!

Your skin may be tough, but it isn't indestructible. A slip of a kitchen knife or a tumble off the curb can cut or tear through the protective layers. Given time, your skin will heal the damage—but in the meantime it hurts like crazy. What can you do?

For starters, of course, you have to stop the bleeding. Once that's done you can take a few steps to speed healing and help the body's natural defenses do their best work. Here's what doctors recommend.

Stop the bleeding. The first thing you need to do for any cut or scrape is to stop the bleeding as soon as possible. Using a piece of gauze or even your hand, apply direct pressure to the wound for five or ten minutes. (If necessary, you can continue applying the pressure for up to thirty minutes.) This will help the blood clot, which should stop the bleeding. If it doesn't stop, you need to see a doctor right away.

Clean it well. Once the bleeding stops, it's important to clean the area thoroughly to prevent infection. Wash it well with soap and water for several minutes. Then apply an antibiotic ointment to prevent infection, and cover the wound with an adhesive bandage or a piece of clean, sterile gauze. The dressing should be snug, but not tight.

Let it breathe. Even though it's a good idea to wear a bandage to prevent infection, it's also important to allow fresh air to reach the wound. Doctors often recommend leaving wounds uncovered, as long as they won't be exposed to grit or anything else that will get inside.

Eat for healing. Your body consumes enormous amounts of nutrients when it's in the midst of healing. Doctors recommend eating plenty of fresh fruit and vegetables. These foods are rich sources of vitamin C and other compounds called bioflavonoids, which have been shown to speed wound healing. Foods that are especially high in these include kiwi, oranges, apples, cranberries, blueberries, strawberries, pineapples, bananas, and grapefruits.

WHEN TO SEE THE DOCTOR

It's easy to treat most cuts and scrapes, but you need to see a doctor if there's a lot of bleeding or if the wound is taking a long time to heal. As a rule, doctors recommend seeking emergency treatment if the blood is spurting (which may mean an artery was cut) or if the wound seems unusually deep. You should also see a doctor if the area gets red or swollen, or if there are streaks of red extending away from the wound. You may need antibiotics to stop an infection.

DANDRUFF

Thanks to the zealous marketing ploys of shampoo manufacturers, dandruff has come to be seen as a disease instead of the entirely natural process that it is.

Everyone gets a little dandruff sometimes. Your scalp, like the rest of your skin, is continually shedding old cells and replacing them with new ones. The life cycle of a skin cell is between two to four weeks, which means old, dead cells—dandruff—are always flaking off. Most of the time you don't even notice them. In some cases, however, the body sheds old skin cells faster than normal. That's when you begin noticing little white flakes in your hair or on the shoulders of your blue blazer.

Doctors aren't sure what causes this acceleration of flaking skin cells, although it may be related to overactive oil glands or possibly a mild fungal infection on the skin. Because the male hormone testosterone plays a role in oil production, dandruff tends to be more common in men than women. It isn't dangerous and it isn't a sign of illness. It can be unsightly, however, which is why people spend millions of dollars every year on products to get rid of the white flakes.

You can't get rid of dandruff entirely, but there are ways to keep the unsightly flakes to a minimum. Here's what dermatologists advise for dandruff sufferers.

Try an oil treatment. When your skin is dry you produce more flaky skin cells than when it's moist and lubricated. That's why experts sometimes recommend massaging a little olive oil into your scalp and leaving it there for about half

52

an hour before showering. The oil will help moisten the scalp and loosen old cells that are getting ready to flake off.

Lather up with a medicated shampoo. Washing your hair often is the best treatment for dandruff because it washes away old skin cells before they become noticeable. Doctors often recommend using medicated dandruff shampoos because they remove skin cells more efficiently than regular shampoos. Look for products containing salicylic acid, selenium, sulfur, or tar.

For dandruff shampoos to work most effectively, it's important to give the medicated ingredients time to work. After lathering, allow the shampoo to stay in your hair for a few minutes before rinsing. This will allow the active ingredients to penetrate the upper layers of skin and help remove old cells. Over-the-counter dandruff shampoos are gentle enough to use regularly, but you'll probably only need to use them for a week or two to get dandruff under control.

Switch brands now and then. Over time your skin can become "immune" to the ingredients in a particular dandruff shampoo. Even if you have a favorite product, it's a good idea to switch brands periodically.

Go easy on the additives. A lot of hair-care products, like mousse, gel, and hair spray, can cause dandruff-like flaking. When you're already having problems with dandruff, these extra flakes will only make the problem worse. It's a good idea to use these products sparingly, and not at all when your dandruff is heaviest.

Try the hat trick. Cold winter air can be extremely drying, which is why many people get more dandruff during the winter months. By wearing a hat you will help keep your skin cells moist and prevent some of the flaking.

53

DEPRESSION

Few things are more discouraging than feeling sad and "down" when everyone else seems to be having a great time. Whether you're simply having a few days of the blues or you've been feeling moody and under the weather for months, depression can be devastating, affecting your relationships, your job, and your life.

Feelings of depression are incredibly common. Experts estimate that ten to twelve million Americans suffer at least occasional bouts of depression. It's twice as common in women, although women are more likely than men to be able to pull themselves out of depression over time. You can't stop depression entirely. After all, life doesn't always go smoothly and there are simply days when you won't want to get out of bed in the morning.

Doctors have found that it's often not the depression itself that's the biggest problem, but how you respond to it. By tackling depression head-on—by staying active, eating right, and doing your best to keep a positive mental attitude—it's often possible to keep it under control or even prevent it entirely.

Get plenty of B vitamins. Researchers have found that people who don't get enough B vitamins, especially vitamin B12, are particularly prone to depression. This can be a real problem in the elderly, since doctors estimate that about one in ten people over age sixty may have mood problems caused by low levels of this vital nutrient. The B vitamins help your body metabolize amino acids, which can help increase the levels of "feel-good" chemicals in the brain.

54

You can get a lot of B vitamins simply by eating a well-rounded, nutritious diet that includes a lot of grains, fruits, and vegetables and that is low in sugars and fats. In addition, doctors often recommend taking a B-complex multivitamin, especially if you're age forty or older.

Take the herbal route. Researchers have found that a number of herbs, such as St. John's Wort, chamomile, and kava kava, can help change your natural chemistry, making you less prone to depression. In fact, European and American doctors have found that St. John's Wort may be as effective as some prescription drugs for treating depression.

The easiest way to use herbs is to buy them in dried, bulk form at natural food stores and brew them up to make a tea. Herbal supplements are also very effective, although you'll want to talk to your doctor to find out what dose will be most effective for you.

Be as active as possible. Regular exercise has been shown to be one of the most powerful anti-depression remedies there are. When you exercise, your body produces large amounts of endorphins, natural chemicals that relieve your feelings of sadness and boost feelings of comfort and well-being. It doesn't take a lot of exercise to release these chemicals. Taking a walk several times a week, riding a bike, or swimming for twenty to thirty minutes may be all it takes to flood your body with these mood-lifters. Most people find that within a week or two of starting an exercise routine they feel happier and more energetic, and sleep better.

Keep in touch with your friends. It's hard to be social when you're feeling down. But spending time with friends is one of the best ways to beat depression. Even if you're just meeting people after work or going to the movies, regular social interactions will help you feel like you're not alone, and this is crucial when you're trying to beat the blues.

55

Write it down. Keeping a journal is an excellent way to stay in touch with your feelings. It can give you a better sense of the types of things that are dragging you down— as well as lifting you up. Sometimes just expressing your emotions will help you feel a whole lot better.

Accept compromise. Many people who are depressed engage in what doctors call "all-or-nothing" thinking, believing everything must go absolutely perfectly. This type of thinking can make you feel as though you're always failing. It's important to recognize that life is almost never all-or-nothing—that there are many shades of gray in everything we do. The more you put things in context, the less likely you'll be to get depressed when things don't go entirely your way. Of course, this is easy to say but sometimes hard to do.

Take inventory of the medicine chest. Many prescription drugs, including some that are taken for high blood pressure, glaucoma, and heart problems, can cause depression in some people. When your mood just doesn't seem to be getting better, make a list of all the medications you're taking and call your doctor. There may be a chemical reason that you're feeling low, and changing medications may be all that's needed to improve your mood again.

WHEN TO SEE THE DOCTOR

Doctors divide depression into two main types. There's "normal" depression, which is simply the blues we all get from time to time. More serious is "clinical" depression, which can make you feel hopeless all the time. When depression is severe and doesn't go away—and you're brooding, sleeping too much, bingeing on food, or generally having trouble coping—it's essential to see a doctor right away. With a combination of therapy and new medications, depression is easier to treat than ever before. But you can't do it on your own. Serious depression always requires professional care.

DIARRHEA

Diarrhea is one of your body's natural defenses. It rushes things through the digestive tract that your body wants to get rid of. Knowing this won't make you feel any better when you're running for the bathroom every ten minutes, but it's important to understand that diarrhea is very efficient at what it does. It's so efficient, in fact, that it rarely lasts more than a day or two—and that definitely should make you feel better.

The bad news, of course, is that diarrhea often comes back—again and again. Doctors estimate that Americans weather some 100 million cases of diarrhea each year. Most come from bacterial or viral infections, although diarrhea can also be caused by food allergies, stress, a sensitivity to milk or other dairy foods, or even as a side effect of medications.

Even though diarrhea may play a protective role, you don't want it to last too long because it can rob your body of essential fluids and nutrients. And of course, it just plain feels awful. Here are a few ways to speed it on its way.

WHEN TO SEE THE DOCTOR

Diarrhea can remove enormous amounts of fluids from your body. If it doesn't stop within a few days it can lead to dehydration, which can be serious if it isn't treated promptly. You should call your doctor whenever diarrhea lasts longer than two or three days, or if it's accompanied by other symptoms, such as blood in the stool, fever, vomiting, or serious abdominal pain.

57

Drink a lot of fluids. To stay healthy, it's essential to replace all the fluids that diarrhea takes out of you. Doctors recommend drinking as much as you can hold—at least eight to twelve glasses of water a day. Sports drinks are even better than water because they contain many essential minerals, called electrolytes, that you need to stay healthy. You can also purchase flavored electrolyte solutions at your local pharmacy.

Give your system a break. It's generally important to eat well to keep up your strength, but when you have diarrhea it's better to eat less to give your digestive tract time to recover. Doctors recommend sticking to a "clear" diet by eating foods such as broth or gelatin. When you're ready to start eating solid foods again, keep it bland for a few days by eating easy-to-digest foods such as rice, bananas, applesauce, and toast. Avoid acidic foods, such as oranges and tomatoes, which can irritate the digestive tract.

Have a little yogurt. Yogurt can be very good for diarrhea if it contains "active" cultures—beneficial bacteria that help aid in digestion. The label will tell you.

Avoid high-fiber foods. When you have diarrhea it's important to eat foods that are easy to digest. Dietary fiber, for all its benefits, isn't digested, which makes it harder for the digestive tract to do its job. Once the diarrhea has run its course, you can start eating a high-fiber diet again.

Take advantage of berries. Blueberries may be the perfect diarrhea-fighting food. They're rich in protein, which your body needs when you're feeling sick. Plus, they contain compounds that may help stop bacteria that can cause diarrhea in the first place.

Take the Mary Poppins prescription. Even if you don't need any help getting the medicine down, a spoonful of sugar can be very helpful when you're fighting diarrhea. Sugar helps the body absorb—rather than eliminate—water, so it can help prevent dehydration.

Ask your doctor about dairy. If you're having diarrhea all the time, you could be sensitive to lactose, a sugar found in milk and other dairy foods. In fact, doctors believe that "lactose intolerance" is a very common cause of diarrhea. You may want to try giving up milk, cheese, and other dairy foods for a few days to see if the problem goes away. Or you can take supplements containing lactase—an enzyme that will help your body digest the lactose in dairy foods.

Get quick relief at the pharmacy. Doctors usually recommend letting diarrhea run its course. But when you have to stop it fast—because you're taking a business trip, for example—you may want to pick up some imodium at the pharmacy. This over-the-counter medication helps prevent the intestines from contracting, which stops diarrhea fast.

EARACHE

It's bad enough that you've gone through two boxes of tissues in one day and your chest feels like it's filled with foam rubber. But now your ears are getting into the act.

Many people get earaches when they have a head cold. The same congestion that makes it hard to breathe can also block the eustachian tube—which runs from the back of the throat to the inner ear. When mucus or pus build up next to the eardrum they can cause excruciating pain. In addition, the insides of the ears provide a perfectly warm, moist environment for bacteria and other organisms to thrive. When

59

you've been swimming or had a head cold, some germs can multiply in the inner ear, causing a painful infection. Your ears are constantly open to the environment, so it's not always easy to prevent problems. But there are many ways to ease the ache so you can rest easily again. Here's how.

WHEN TO SEE THE DOCTOR

Most ear infections will clear up on their own, but sometimes the infection sticks around, getting more and more painful. When a "minor" earache is starting to feel major, or if there's pus or a discharge coming from inside the ear, you need to call your doctor right away. You probably have an infection, and you may need antibiotics to get rid of it.

Warm it up. The quickest way to ease an earache is to place a hot water bottle or a heating pad (set to a comfortable temperature) on top of your ear. Better yet, cover your ear with a towel that's been moistened with warm water. The combination of heat and moisture can be very soothing. As a bonus, the heat will help melt ear wax, which could be contributing to the congestion.

Put garlic to work. Recent evidence suggests that squeezing a clove of garlic and putting a few drops in your ear will help kill bacteria that are causing the pain. In fact, researchers suspect that garlic may be even more effective than some prescription antibiotics.

Give it the oil treatment. Putting a few drops of mineral oil in your ear can help dissolve wax and ease the pain momentarily. Mineral oil will be most effective when it's warm, so heat a little oil in a tablespoon, then let it cool to about body temperature before putting it in your ear.

Fight back with echinacea. This traditional healing remedy, available at health food stores and some grocers, has been shown to stimulate the immune system so it's better able to fight the infection. Keep some echinacea handy in your kitchen or bathroom cupboard, so as soon as ear pain strikes, you can take them as needed. You can also buy echinacea in a tincture form, which is added to hot water to make a tea. Echinacea also works well for colds, which could be the source of earaches.

Clear out the wax. It's normal for the ears to produce a little wax, which helps trap grit and debris before they get into the inner ear. When you have too much ear wax, however, it can change the pressure inside your ear, causing earaches. For helpful tips on getting rid of ear wax, see the Ear Wax chapter on page 62.

Try a decongestant. Because earaches often are caused by congestion, you may want to drop by the pharmacy and pick up a decongestant. These products will reduce congestion in the sinuses and throat, relieving pressure in the ears. Be sure to follow all label directions and warnings carefully, of course.

Take flight precautions. Air travel is fast and convenient, but it isn't without drawbacks. When you soar above sea level the pressure inside the ears changes, which often causes earaches. Flying can be especially uncomfortable if you already have a cold or congestion. To reduce the discomfort, bring along some gum. Chewing helps reduce the pressure that causes the pain.

Practice "sound" advice. The ears really aren't designed to tolerate loud noise. Studies have shown that anything louder than normal conversation or heavy traffic can gradually damage the inner ear, causing hearing loss as well as pain. When you're going to be in a noisy place—a rock concert, for example, or in the yard with a chain saw—wearing ear plugs will help prevent earaches and long-term damage.

61

EAR WAX

The insides of your ears are filled with very tiny, delicate instruments that make it possible for you to enjoy everything from the crash of cymbals to the soft murmur of a mountain stream. To protect this sensitive area, the ears have tiny glands that produce wax that lines the ear canal. Ear wax, along with small hair follicles, traps dust and debris before it reaches the inner ear. Over time, the wax then migrates to the outer ear where it's easy to remove with the tip of a handkerchief.

Some people, however, produce more ear wax than the ear can easily get rid of. Over time the wax begins to accumulate. If the opening leading to the eardrum gets blocked, you may lose some of your hearing. Too much ear wax also can be painful because it can cause pressure changes inside the inner ear.

It's usually not difficult to get ear wax under control. Here's what you need to do.

WHEN TO SEE THE DOCTOR

Ear wax can be a serious problem when you produce too much of it. If you can actually see excess wax in the outer part of the ear, of if your hearing seems to be getting worse or you're hearing ringing or other noises, you need to see your doctor. There could be something wrong in the inner ear that will need to be corrected to prevent additional problems.

62

Soften it up. When your body is producing a lot of ear wax, it can get nearly rock-hard, making it difficult to remove. To soften the wax, put a few drops of mineral oil, baby oil, or glycerin in your ear with an eyedropper, then roll your head around to let the oil soak in. If you do this twice a day for several days, the wax will get much softer and will start moving toward the outside of the ear, where it's easier to remove.

Bubble it away. Another way to soften ear wax is to fill an eyedropper with hydrogen peroxide and squirt it into your ears. Let it sit and bubble for a few minutes, then drain your ear by tilting your head to the side. The bubbles will help dislodge small particles of wax, which will drain out with the fluid.

Add a little heat. Just like wax in a candle, ear wax melts when it gets warm. Resting your ear on top of a hot water bottle or a heating pad (set to a comfortable temperature) will warm up the ear canal and soften or even melt the wax. Keep your head tilted down, which will allow the wax to flow toward the outside of your ear.

Give your ears a good washing. Once you've loosened the ear wax, fill a three-ounce rubber bulb syringe with water that's about body temperature (98.6° F). With your head tilted down, pull your outer ear out a little to straighten the ear canal. Then gently squirt some water into the canal. The water will help break up ear wax and float it along the canal toward the outside of your ear. When you're done, dry your ear with a towel and squirt a little bit of rubbing alcohol inside. Then tilt your head so the fluid drains out. The rubbing alcohol will help dry the ear canal, reducing the risk of infection. And, it will help kill any infection-causing organisms that may be present.

Put on the pressure. According to acupressurists, applying pressure to the fourth finger of the hand on the side with the blocked-up ear will help relieve pain that may accompany waxy build-ups. Then gently massage the soft area behind the ear, near the jaw.

Clean your ears with care. When ear wax starts building up, many people go after it with a cotton swab—and inadvertently push the wax deeper inside. Eventually it can form a hard little plug that can be almost impossible to get out. Doctors recommend cleaning the outside of your ears only—not with a cotton swab, but with the tip of a washcloth that's been moistened in a little water. This will keep your ears clean without pushing additional wax where it isn't meant to go.

EYESTRAIN AND DRY EYES

In terms of eyestrain, our ancestors had it easy. Today, we spend hours every day staring into computer monitors or TV screens, squinting through dirty windshields, or simply opening our eyes every morning in a world that's full of smoke and smog. As a result, our eyes often are tired and dry.

WHEN TO SEE THE DOCTOR

If your eyes are dry and sore, and you have other symptoms like a dry mouth, you should call your doctor right away. There are a number of illnesses, including arthritis and lupus, that can cause the eyes to get tired and irritated. Don't assume that dry eyes are "merely" an eye problem. There may be something else going on as well.

To give your eyes a break while keeping them moist and lubricated, here's what doctors advise.

Bat your eyelids. Your eyelids are like windshield wipers. Every time you blink they spread a soothing layer of lubrication across the surfaces of the eyes. When your eyes are getting tired, blinking your eyes several times will give quick relief. As a bonus, blinking helps remove dust or grit from the eyes before it causes irritation.

Cover your eyes. To soothe the eyes, do what professional massage therapists do: Rub your hands together to warm them up, then place the heels of your palms over your eyes for a few seconds. The warmth from your hands will quickly penetrate into the eyes, making them feel rested and relaxed.

Give nature a hand. When your eyes are unusually dry, put in a few drops of artificial tears. Sold in pharmacies, these "re-wetting drops" will help remove debris while providing soothing relief. You can use artificial tears whenever your eyes are feeling dry and tired.

Keep them cool. Many people have found that putting slices of cool cucumber over the eyes can be very soothing. Or you can simply cover your eyes with a cool compress. Wet a towel in cool water, wring it out, and place it over your eyes for about five minutes.

Give your eyes a break. Most eyestrain is caused by overuse—from staring at the computer screen, for example, or driving long distances. Doctors recommend taking a "vision break" once an hour or so. You don't have to stop what you're doing—just focus on something else for a few minutes, preferably something in the distance. Then close your eyes and relax for a moment. Simply resting your eyes now and then will make a big difference in stopping strain and soreness.

65

FATIGUE

Maybe you're fighting to keep your eyes open even before lunch time. Or perhaps you're going to bed earlier each night but are still waking up feeling like you haven't had enough sleep. Or maybe you simply don't have the energy to do the things you'd like to do.

Welcome to modern life. Doctors agree that our hectic pace—the endless meetings, rushing home to care for the children, and staying up a little too late at night—is taking its toll. People are feeling more tired than ever before, and there doesn't seem to be any relief in sight.

You can't turn the clock back to a simpler time, of course. But there are ways you can boost your energy and restore your enjoyment of life. Here's what experts recommend.

WHEN TO SEE THE DOCTOR

While fatigue is often caused by nothing worse than a lack of sleep, it can also be a sign of other, underlying problems, including diabetes, anemia, hormonal imbalances, or even chronic fatigue syndrome. If you're tired all the time and it seems to be getting worse, you need to get a checkup. Your doctor will probably do a variety of tests, including blood tests, to figure out what's going on and what you need to do.

Make sure the well doesn't run dry. When you're busy all day it's easy to forget to drink enough water. When you don't get enough fluids, cells throughout your body, including in the brain, begin to run dry, which can sap your energy. Don't wait until you're feeling thirsty, because your body's "thirst-sensor" doesn't always work efficiently. Doctors say to drink at least eight glasses a day.

Incidentally, don't count coffee or cola toward your daily total. These drinks contain caffeine, which is a diuretic—meaning it actually removes more fluids from your body than it puts in. If you do drink coffee or other beverages with caffeine, you need to drink even more water to keep yourself hydrated.

See the light. When winter arrives and days get shorter, many people start feeling tired and fatigued. Studies have shown, however, that you can give your energy a boost by getting more sunlight. Even if you only get outside for an hour or two a day, the extra light may help put extra zip in your mood.

Shake things up. Sometimes it seems like every day is the same. We go to work, go home, cook dinner, go to bed. It's no wonder that we sometimes feel a little tired and unmotivated. Doctors agree that one of the best things you can do to fight fatigue is to put more variety into your life. Going for walks, taking adult-education classes, or simply reading some new books will help you feel more motivated and energized by life.

Add some color to your life. Studies have shown that people who spend their time in dark houses with dull, muted colors tend to have less energy than those who are surrounded by visual "zip"—bright reds, soothing greens, or vibrant yellows. Even if you don't feel like painting your house, it's a good idea to liven up your surroundings.

Eat for energy. Many people can make themselves feel stronger and more energetic simply by eating a better diet. Unlike foods that are high in fat, which are hard to digest and tend to sap your energy, fruits, vegetables, and carbohydrates can help you feel more energized.

Ban the big meals. If you work in an office you know that the lowest-energy time of day is right after lunch, when just

67

about everyone is nodding off. This is due in part to the body's natural need for rest. But studies have shown that people who eat four or five small meals a day tend to have more energy than those who eat two or three big meals. Try to eat a good-sized breakfast, one or two healthy snacks during the day (but not a big lunch), and a good meal at supper. Eating frequent smaller meals helps keep your metabolism burning steadily, rather than working hard all at once. And eating regularly helps keep blood-sugar levels steady, which can be very powerful in fighting fatigue.

Get as much exercise as you can. Even when your energy is so low you don't want to lace your tennis shoes, it's worth making yourself stay active. Exercise helps burn off stress and frustration, while at the same time increases the amount of energizing chemicals in your body. Studies have shown that people who exercise regularly report feeling more ambitious, optimistic, and energetic.

Put relaxation on your calendar. Relieving stress is a skill that should be taught in school. Most of us have a hard time making time for rest and relaxation—and we pay for it in lost energy. One of the best ways to recharge your batteries is to put aside a little time each day to do something you truly enjoy—playing with your dog, shopping, or even getting a massage. Taking a break from life's stresses gives your body and mind time to recover, which will help you feel stronger the rest of the time.

Get to bed earlier. It's obvious advice, but a lot of us walk around like zombies simply because we try to squeeze too much out of each day. Going to bed an hour or two earlier on a regular basis will help ensure that you get the sleep you need—the sleep you're probably not getting enough of now.

FEVER

They don't feel good, but fevers are your body's tool for waging war on bacteria and other germs. These microorganisms are able to thrive only at certain temperatures. When you're sick with a cold, the flu, or another kind of infection, your body turns up the thermostat. As you get hotter, the germs are no longer able to reproduce—which means you get better faster.

Of course, knowing that a fever is good for you doesn't make you feel any better. (Root canals are also good for you, and you know how much you look forward to them.) But it's helpful to realize that most fevers don't last very long, and by the time your temperature starts dropping you're well on the road to recovery.

For mild fevers, doctors usually recommend letting them run their course, although you may want to take aspirin or acetaminophen, which will lower your temperature a bit and make you feel more comfortable. (Children with fever should never be given aspirin because of the risk of Reye's syndrome, a serious neurological disorder.) Here are a few additional ways to turn the temperature down.

Drink plenty of fluids. Just as your car's radiator may burn off extra water when it's running hot, people with fevers also burn more water. To replace the fluids that fevers take out, it's important to drink at least eight to twelve glasses of water a day. You may want to drink a sports drink like Gatorade, as well. These drinks contain electrolytes—minerals that can help your body work more efficiently. Electrolyte drinks are also available in your local pharmacy.

69

WHEN TO SEE THE DOCTOR

Adults and children have thermostats that are set at different levels. For adults, any fever over 101 degrees that lasts more than three days is potentially serious and should be treated by a physician. Children tend to run a little hotter. If a child has a fever of 103 degrees or higher, or a lower temperature that lasts for more than three days, you should call your doctor right away. For children under one year, however, a fever over 101 degrees could be serious and a doctor visit is recommended. You should also call your doctor if a fever is accompanied by other symptoms, such as diarrhea, sore throat, or a stomachache.

Take a long soak. Just because you're hot on the inside doesn't mean you have to be hot and sweaty on the outside. When you feel a fever coming on, fill the bathtub with lukewarm water and settle in for a long soak. It will help lower your body temperature so you feel a bit more comfortable. Don't soak in cold water, however. That can cool you off too much and may make you worse.

Spend some time in bed. A fever means that your body is using up a lot of energy fighting an infection. Getting extra rest will help ensure that your body has enough energy left over to do what's important—stimulating the immune system to help you recover.

FLATULENCE

It's uncomfortable. It's embarrassing. And there's no way to prevent it. Flatulence may be socially unacceptable, but it's a natural by-product of digestion. The average person, in fact, passes gas eight to twenty times a day.

Even though you can't stop gas entirely, there are ways to reduce its frequency. Here's how.

Pour a cup of tea. Herbal teas have been used for thousands of years to aid digestion. Natural healers often recommend mint, sage, or anise tea for digestive complaints, including gas.

Drink milk with caution. It doesn't bother everyone, but some people have trouble digesting a sugar (called lactose) in milk, cheese, and other dairy foods. This condition, called lactose intolerance, is a very common cause of gas. You may get some relief simply by cutting back on dairy foods. Many people, however, have to give them up entirely. Another alternative is to take supplements containing lactase, an enzyme that helps people digest the lactose found in dairy foods.

Stick with the real thing. Sugar may not be the best thing for your waistline, but it's better than artificial sweeteners when it comes to your digestion. Doctors estimate that up to one-half of Americans have trouble digesting sorbitol and mannitol, two common artificial sweeteners that are used in sugar-free foods, such as candies and gum. In fact, the amount of sorbitol in just five sticks of gum may cause gas and diarrhea in some people.

Breathe slowly. Many people routinely swallow large amounts of air, especially while eating. That extra air has

71

to go somewhere—and out it goes, many times a day. To make sure that the air you breathe goes into your lungs and not into your stomach, doctors recommend breathing slowly through your nose rather than gulping air through your mouth. Chewing food more slowly and not chomping away at your gum also can reduce the amount of air that gets inside. Some experts suggest giving up carbonated drinks, as well, because all those bubbles may cause flatulence too.

Experiment with your diet. If you find yourself constantly battling flatulence, do some experimenting to find the cause. Maybe it's not the salad, but the radishes that are causing problems. Perhaps it's not the pasta and sauce, but the extra garlic you've added. By becoming a food sleuth, you'll learn to eat strategically to avoid gas attacks.

Ease into fiber. Even though dietary fiber is very good for your health, it can cause flatulence in people who aren't yet used to it. If you've just begun adding more fruits, vegetables, and other high-fiber foods to your diet, do yourself a favor and make the additions slowly. If you give your body time to get used to this new substance, you're less likely to have a problem with gas.

Eat sitting up. When you're having problems with gas, don't take your meals while reclining on the couch. Reclining or slouching when you eat can put bends in the digestive tract that make it hard for gas to escape upward—so it goes out the other way. Sitting straight, on the other hand, allows gas in the stomach to exit in a less embarrassing fashion—through the mouth.

72

Talk to your pharmacist. There are a number of over-the-counter products that can help prevent gas. One you may want to try is called Beano. It contains an enzyme that breaks down sugars in the digestive tract, which helps to prevent gas from forming. Or you might want to try products containing simethicone, which can help break up gas bubbles in the digestive tract.

FLU

At first it feels like a cold: runny nose, dry eyes, maybe a cough. But within a few days you'll know that this is no common cold. The flu virus can be especially virulent, causing fever, chills, sore throat, and fatigue. In addition, your muscles may be so sore that you feel like you fell off a ten-story building.

The flu virus usually makes its rounds during the cold months, although it's possible to get it in the summer and spring. There are three categories of flu viruses: Type A, which is the most serious, and Types B and C, which aren't as common and usually won't make you as sick. When doctors talk about "the flu," it's the Type A influenza virus.

The easiest way to prevent the flu is to get a flu shot every year. If you're already sick, however, what you need is fast relief. Here's what doctors recommend.

WHEN TO SEE THE DOCTOR

Most people are able to weather a bout with the flu without serious problems. But this virus can be dangerous for the elderly, as well as for people with weakened immune systems or other health problems. If you get the flu and also are having chest pains or difficulty breathing, you need to call your doctor right away.

Buy a new toothbrush. The virus that causes the flu can live for days on a wet toothbrush. What this means is that every time you brush your teeth, more of the bugs get into your bloodstream, causing you to get sick all over again. Doctors advise tossing your old toothbrush a few days after you get the flu and replacing it with a new one, which you can use for the duration of the illness.

Wash your hands often. It's not only your toothbrush that can transmit the flu virus. Touching your mouth, eyes, or nose with your hands also can put more of the germs in your system. During flu season it's a good idea to wash your hands several times a day with soap and water. This is especially important if you work in an office with other people, who may pass their flu germs to you.

Humidify the air. One reason the flu is so common in the winter months is that the cold, dry air removes moisture from protective membranes in your nose and throat, making it easier for germs to get in. Plugging in a humidifier will fill the air with water droplets. These droplets help keep your mucus membranes moist, so they're better able to trap infection-causing germs.

Drink lots of water. A bout with the flu can rob your body of enormous amounts of water. Drinking eight or more glasses of water a day will help keep your mucus membranes moist and help relieve dry eyes, sore throat, and other common flu symptoms.

FORGETFULNESS

Do you have a secret suspicion that your reading glasses scamper away whenever you put them down? Or that someone is sneaking out to the parking lot and moving your car from where you left it?

No one's memory is perfect, and as we get older our memories tend to get less perfect every day. Forgetting things now and then probably does not mean that you are getting Alzheimer's disease. In most cases, it simply means that your brain isn't able to retain as many of the little daily details as it used to.

Like any other part of your body, your brain needs exercise in order to work most efficiently. In addition, there are a lot of simple strategies that will help you remember things even when your brain isn't cooperating. Here's what doctors advise.

Set a schedule. Immanuel Kant, who is often considered the greatest philosopher of all time, kept a schedule so precise that town folks could set their clocks by his afternoon walks. If keeping a schedule freed up Kant's mind enough to revolutionize philosophy, think what it can do for you.

Doctors often recommend that people with memory problems do all of their routines according to a schedule: Wake at the same time, wind your watch first thing in the morning, water the plants every Friday, and so on. By ingraining a schedule into your memory, you'll free yourself from having to remember those 1,001 details that might otherwise get overlooked.

Try the Orient express. Some memory loss is caused by poor blood flow to the brain. Since ancient times, the Chinese have used leaves from the ginkgo biloba tree, believed to be one of the oldest trees on the earth, to treat cerebral and cardiovascular conditions because of its talent for increasing blood flow to the brain and other parts of the body. Ginkgo can be purchased in capsule form at many groceries and drugstores, as well as at natural or health food stores.

Cut down on fat. Did you ever get that sluggish feeling after a meal, when you just can't think, let alone remember small details? A fatty diet slows down blood flow to your brain, increasing forgetfulness. Try to cut down on fat in general, and replace products such as butter with unsaturated oils such as safflower oil.

Absorb the details. We live in a busy world with zillions of details zipping by every day. It's impossible to always remember them all. What you can do, however, is make a conscious effort to remember the details that matter. Practice observing things around you. Mentally narrate what you're seeing, doing, and experiencing. With practice, you'll find that you're remembering more and more things with less effort. In fact, you'll begin noticing all of these details without even being aware you're doing it.

Repeat the facts. How many times have you heard someone's name and forgotten it a second later? Here's a trick for remembering things better: Repeat them. Mentally repeating names, dates, and other details helps cement them in your mind, making them easier to recall later on.

76

Create memory links. Memory experts have clever techniques to help people remember, called mnemonic devices. These are simply mind games to help you associate the thing you want to remember with something else that's nearby and familiar. Linking the two makes them much easier to remember. Mnemonic devices often are rhymes or mental pictures. Suppose, for example, you need to pick up eggs at the store. The mnemonic device might be "I won't forget to walk my legs over to the store." Or perhaps you just met someone named Paul, who happens to be six feet tall. To remember his name you might tell yourself, "He's tall Paul."

Create memory zones. If you're constantly misplacing those eyeglasses or keys, designate one area in your home as an "easy memory zone"—the one place you'll always put things you know you're in danger of losing. It could be the top of the refrigerator, a table in the living room, or anywhere else. As long as you always use it, you'll never have to search for your car keys again.

Keep your mind active. Many of us stop exercising our minds at about the same time we leave school—and that's a mistake. The brain needs constant stimulation to stay strong and agile. So set aside a little time for *mindercise*. Take up Scrabble or other word games. Read. Do crossword puzzles. Engage in lively conversation, or tune in to interesting television and radio programs. Anything you can do to keep your mind active will make it stronger—and that's the best way to forget about forgetting.

WHEN TO SEE THE DOCTOR

Forgetting where you parked your car is forgetfulness. Forgetting that you own a car—or constantly forgetting how to get to the parking lot—is something altogether different. Doctors have a simple rule for determining if memory problems are serious: If forgetfulness is jeopardizing your safety or the safety of others, or if you can't remember obvious details like the year, the name of the president, or entire chunks of your past, there's certainly something wrong and you should see your doctor right away.

GINGIVITIS

It's a scary thought, but doctors estimate there are several hundred kinds of bacteria that consider a person's mouth their home. They camp out on your teeth, on and under the tongue, and along (and inside) the gums. As the years go by, the constant bacterial onslaught can cause the gums to swell, redden, and bleed. Doctors call this condition gingivitis, better known as gum disease.

Gingivitis isn't particularly serious in the early stages. If you don't stop it right away, however, it can lead to a more serious condition called periodontitis, which can actually weaken the teeth, making them more likely to loosen.

The one good thing about gingivitis is that it's very easy to reverse. Flossing and brushing your teeth every day will remove build-ups of plaque, a thin, bacteria-laden film that covers the teeth and may lead to gum disease. To save your smile and keep your teeth looking bright, here's what dentists advise.

Give your teeth a good brushing. It was good advice when you heard it from your parents, and it's still the best way to prevent gum disease. If you brush your teeth and gums every day you will remove plaque and bacteria before they have a chance to cause gingivitis. Don't try to finish the whole job in ten seconds. For brushing to be effective you have to hit every tooth, from the front as well as the back. While you're at it, take a few seconds to brush along the gum line. By taking your time—dentists advise brushing for two or three minutes—you'll virtually eliminate the plaque that can cause problems later on.

Don't forget the tongue. If you don't brush it every day, your tongue can provide safe haven for millions of infection-causing bacteria. You don't have to spend a lot of time on it. Just giving your tongue a quick brushing will remove bacteria as well as food particles.

Put the floss to work. It's not the most exciting activity, but flossing your teeth will remove build-ups of plaque and bacteria between your teeth where a brush can't reach, and will strengthen your gums. It doesn't really matter what kind of floss you use—mint-flavored, flat or thin, they all work about the same. Use the kind that feels most comfortable to you, and use it every day.

Use a pick. If you're not able to floss every day, dentists recommend using those flat, wooden toothpicks you can buy at pharmacies. The picks are designed to fit between your teeth and along the gum line. They will remove plaque and bacteria that your brush leaves behind.

Add a little force. A high-tech version of the toothpick is the Water-Pic. This little gadget fires a jet of water between your teeth and into the gum line, floating away particles that brushing doesn't get. You can buy Water-Pics at pharmacies and many department stores.

Turn on the power. Studies have shown that an electric toothbrush can remove more plaque than brushing manually does. Ask your dentist what brand and style will work best for you.

Brush after eating sticky foods. Sugar isn't the best thing for your teeth, but it isn't the demon dentists once thought it was. A more serious threat for your teeth are sticky treats. Things like chocolate and caramel stick to the surfaces of the teeth, making it easy for bacteria to stick around. You don't have to give up your favorite snacks. Just be sure to brush your teeth thoroughly after eating them.

79

Get some help from vitamin C. Research has shown that getting plenty of vitamin C in your diet as well as taking supplements can help bleeding gums heal more quickly. You can get plenty of this healthful nutrient by enjoying citrus fruits (or drinking orange juice) and green, leafy vegetables. If you're not getting enough vitamin C in your diet, you may want to take a 500-milligram supplement once a day, dentists say.

See red. Not sure if you're taking good care of your teeth? You may want to ask your dentist for those tiny tablets that will stain accumulations of plaque with red dye. They're a great way to see how effective your brushing really is.

WHEN TO SEE THE DOCTOR (OR DENTIST)

Gum disease isn't serious when it first begins, but over time it can damage the gums and even the supporting bone underneath. Signs of serious gum disease include breath that's always bad, "longer" teeth (a result of shrinking gums), gums that keep bleeding, or pus in between the teeth and gums. If you notice any of these signs, it's essential to call your dentist right away.

HANGOVER

Through the ages there have been invented nearly as many hangover remedies as there are varieties of mixed drinks. Most of them, unfortunately, don't work.

If you've ever made too many trips to the punch bowl, you're all too familiar with the pounding head, queasy stomach, dry mouth, and other miserable symptoms that accompany hangovers. But even though people have been getting hangovers for thousands of years, doctors aren't sure exactly what they are or what's the best remedy. But they do have some ideas. Here are a few things you may want to try.

Have a little honey. Honey contains large amounts of a natural sugar called fructose, which is burned very quickly by the body. By putting your metabolism in high gear, it will help your body burn off the alcohol faster.

Pass up the coffee. When you prop up your tired eyes, the coffee pot is probably the first thing you're going to reach for. When you have a hangover, however, your body is already dehydrated. Coffee is a diuretic, which means it removes more fluids from your body than it puts in—and that's the last thing you need when you're coping with a hangover.

Take some vitamin C. Evidence suggests that vitamin C can help the body get rid of alcohol more quickly. Taking about 500 milligrams of vitamin C or eating vitamin C-rich foods like oranges or grapefruit may be one of the best ways to relieve the hangover blues.

Keep your stomach full. When the crowd is partying hearty, it's a good idea to have some food in your stomach. High-protein foods are especially good because they take a long time to digest. Keeping food in your system will help slow the absorption of alcohol and also provide essential nutrients that may help counter the effects the next day.

Avoid salty foods. There's a good reason bartenders often put out bowls of pretzels and beer nuts. Salty foods make you drink more, so you'll spend more money. What's good

81

for the bar's bottom line, however, isn't so good for your body. All that salt can dry you out, which can make hangovers even worse.

Top off your tank before going to bed. After a night of drinking alcohol, it's a good idea to drink a few glasses of water as well. Being dehydrated is one of the main reasons hangovers feel so awful. Drinking water before bed and as soon as you get up in the morning will go a long way toward making you feel better.

HEADACHES

The kids are yelling. The phone's ringing. Your husband's complaining about work and the dog just ate the roast. This is more than just tension. You feel like your head's in a vise and it's getting tighter all the time.

Your body responds to stress in a lot of different ways, and one of the most common—and painful—is headaches. Studies show that as many as forty million Americans see their doctors every year for headache pain, and about 90 percent of those headaches are caused by tension. It's no wonder that Americans spend up to $400 million a year on over-the-counter pain pills like aspirin and ibuprofen.

82

It's not only tension that causes "tension headaches." Despite the name, this type of headache can be caused by anything from muscle tension in the neck and shoulders to eyestrain, allergies, too much coffee, and jaw problems.

(Migraines are a different type of headache altogether. For more information on migraines, see page 108.) Any one of these problems, or a combination of them, can cause a head-pounding, jaw-clenching headache.

There's no way to prevent headaches entirely, but there are many things you can do to keep the pain from driving you out of your head. Here's how.

WHEN TO SEE THE DOCTOR

When headache pain strikes, everything else in your life comes to a standstill. Most headaches will go away on their own within a few hours, or at most, a few days. If your head keeps hurting, however, and you have other symptoms like nausea, dizziness, or blurred vision, you should call your doctor. You should also call your doctor if you're having headaches as well as jaw pain, or if there are clicking or popping sounds in the jaw. These could be signs of a jaw problem called TMD, or temporomandibular joint disorder, which can be serious without treatment. (For more information on TMD, see page 161.)

Keep a cool head. If you act quickly, applying cold may stop a headache by constricting throbbing blood vessels and reducing inflammation that can lead to pain. The easiest approach is to put some ice cubes in a plastic bag, wrap that in a towel and apply it where you hurt the most. Hold the ice in place for fifteen or twenty minutes. If you're still hurting later on, you can repeat the treatment every few hours.

But warm up your muscles. Since many headaches are caused by tense muscles in the neck and shoulders, applying a heating pad or hot water bottle can be very helpful. Or simply take a hot bath or a long, steamy shower. When your muscles begin to relax, your headache should feel better, too.

Give your eyes a break. Headaches are often caused by nothing more than eyestrain—especially when you've been spending time in front of the computer or the television.

83

Take a few minutes to give your eyes some rest—simply closing them for a few minutes can help relieve the pain. Or soak a towel in cool water, wring it out, and drape it over your eyes for a few minutes.

Cut back on coffee. The caffeine in coffee can cause blood vessels in your head to contract and then dilate, putting pressure on tender nerves. If you suspect that coffee may be part of the problem, switch to decaffeinated tea for a few days to see if things improve.

But sip a little coffee when you take an aspirin. Aspirin is one of the best headache remedies you can find. To make it even more effective, wash it down with a little bit of coffee or cola. Researchers have found that caffeine works with aspirin to make it act more efficiently.

Take advantage of massage. Rubbing your neck, shoulders, and the base of your skull can quickly relax muscle tension, which may be all you need to stop a headache. The most relaxing massage, of course, is one that's given by your spouse or a friend. But you can always do it yourself. Your muscles don't care who gives the massage, as long as it helps relieve some of the tension.

Know what you're eating. There are many foods and ingredients in foods that can cause headaches in some people. Monosodium glutamate (MSG), for example, often used in Asian restaurants, is one of the worst offenders. Many restaurants are happy to prepare your meal without MSG, if you put in a request. Chemicals found in processed foods and smoked meats may also cause headaches. Even red wine can be a problem for some people. So the next time a headache strikes, think about what you've been eating lately. There could be a connection.

HEARTBURN

It's Thanksgiving, the family is gathered, and your dear Aunt Gladys is making sure everyone gets enough to eat. "An extra serving of turkey? Here's a little more stuffing. Did you say you wanted pumpkin pie? Oh, you want the pecan pie. Let me cut you a little slice—no, bigger than that."

Then the dishes are cleared and everyone stretches out in front of the TV—and you can almost hear the flames of heartburn crackling away.

Heartburn wouldn't be a problem if it only occurred after overindulging. But for some people it happens all the time, and it can be extremely uncomfortable.

Despite the name, heartburn has nothing to do with the heart. It occurs when acid in the stomach, instead of staying put, splashes upstream into the esophagus, the tube that connects the mouth to the stomach. While the stomach is designed to withstand acid, the esophagus isn't. Each splash of acid literally scorches the delicate lining of the esophagus. That's what causes the "burn" of heartburn.

WHEN TO SEE THE DOCTOR

If you suffer heartburn daily or several times a week, or if you sometimes have chest pain or a tight, uncomfortable feeling in your chest, call your doctor immediately. The pain caused by heartburn is very similar to the pain caused by real heart problems, including heart attacks. Don't take chances if you aren't sure. Get to a doctor or the emergency room right away.

85

The body normally does a good job of keeping acid where it belongs. There's a tight little ring of muscle at the base of the esophagus that opens to let food into the stomach, then snaps shut to keep acid from surging upstream. In some people, however, the muscle either gets weak or opens and closes at the wrong time, causing heartburn.

Heartburn is rarely serious and can easily be treated at home with a few simple changes.

Wash away the acid. One of the best ways to stop heartburn fast is simply to drink a glass of water. This helps dilute and wash away acid in the esophagus before it has a chance to burn. In fact, drinking water with meals makes heartburn much less likely to occur.

Avoid high-fat foods. Studies have shown that chocolate, French fries, and other high-fat foods can cause the protective muscle in the esophagus to lose its grip, allowing stomach acid to squirt upward.

Skip the breath mints. Peppermint and spearmint may freshen your breath, but they can also feed the fires of heartburn by weakening the "valve" in the esophagus. Smoking does the same thing, so having an after-dinner cigarette can "burn" in more ways than one.

Eat a little less. It doesn't take a holiday feast to cause heartburn. Any time you put a lot of food into the stomach, acid levels rise, making it much more likely to splash upstream. Eating smaller meals more often will help keep acid levels in the stomach low and away from the esophagus.

Give yourself a raise. When you lie down after eating, gravity works against you, making it easier for acid in the stomach to enter the esophagus. Sitting upright for a few hours after meals will help keep the acid where it belongs. Some people find that propping themselves up with pillows when they sleep or raising the head of the bed can also help prevent heartburn.

Consider a diet. When you're overweight there's a lot more pressure on the abdomen, which can cause the muscle in the esophagus to lose its grip.

Schedule your midnight snacks for 8 p.m. When you eat late at night, the stomach produces acids that may linger long past bedtime. Then, when you lie down, the acid is much more likely to creep upstream, causing heartburn and keeping you awake at night. It's a good idea not to eat anything within a few hours of your bedtime.

Check your medicines. A number of prescription drugs, including birth control pills, antihistamines, and heart medications, have been known to weaken the muscle in the esophagus. If you're having heartburn, ask your doctor if medications may be responsible—and if changing drugs might help.

HEMORRHOIDS

This is one condition you probably won't hear your friends discussing at a holiday party—but it's a good bet many of them have occasionally suffered from this problem. Hemorrhoids are very common. Doctors estimate that a majority of Americans get these pesky irritants at one time or another.

Hemorrhoids are veins in the anus, which, instead of moving blood smoothly, get distended and filled with blood. When the blood doesn't flow, the veins gradually swell, like a water balloon. Eventually they get large enough that you start to feel them—and that feeling can be very uncomfortable.

Hemorrhoids usually occur when you strain to have a bowel movement. The increased pressure caused by straining causes the veins to weaken, get flabby, and, then, to swell. Because hemorrhoids are filled with blood, you may notice blood in the toilet bowl or on the toilet paper. When you don't know what's causing it, blood from that area can be very frightening indeed.

The truth is, hemorrhoids are rarely serious, and will usually go away on their own. When they're painful or itchy, however, you're going to want fast relief. Here are a few things that can help.

WHEN TO SEE THE DOCTOR

It's very common for hemorrhoids to bleed, and this isn't considered a problem. Unfortunately, there are a number of other conditions that also cause rectal bleeding, such as polyps and colon cancer. Since it's impossible to know at home what's causing the bleeding, it's important to call your doctor when you first see red. He may recommend that you have a series of tests that will reveal whether or not anything is wrong inside the intestine. Most of the time there won't be. But when it comes to cancer, fast action is essential, so don't wait before calling for help.

Call on the witch. To relieve the itching and burning of hemorrhoids, doctors often recommend applying a little witch hazel. This will quickly cool the area so you feel more comfortable. For extra relief, some people cool the witch hazel first by storing it in the refrigerator.

88

Put water to work. Perhaps the easiest home remedy for hemorrhoids is simply to sit in a warm bath several times a day. The warm water will help relax the anal muscle and improve circulation, which will help hemorrhoids heal.

Don't add bath oils or salts to the water, however, because this may increase the irritation.

Add some lubrication. Spreading a little petroleum jelly on hemorrhoids will help protect the tender skin. Many doctors believe it works as well as special hemorrhoid creams and ointments, and it's much less expensive.

Take advantage of fiber. Foods that are high in dietary fiber make the stools softer and easier to pass. This is important because the less you strain to have a bowel movement, the less likely hemorrhoids are to form. A quick way to get more fiber is to pick up some psyllium at the drugstore. This natural ingredient is found in products such as Metamucil, and it's an excellent way to make stools softer.

Drink a lot of water. Your intestines need a lot of fluid to work smoothly and with a minimum of irritation. Drinking eight to twelve glasses of water a day will provide plenty of lubrication as well as make the stools softer and, therefore, easier to pass.

Check your weight. People who are overweight have a higher risk for hemorrhoids because the extra pounds exert more pressure on the anal area, making hemorrhoids more likely to form. In some cases, losing weight will cause your hemorrhoids to disappear, as well.

HICCUPS

Hiccups are one of life's mysteries. Some people get them all the time and others hardly ever do. They don't serve any purpose. And they usually come out of nowhere. One minute you're carrying on a normal conversation, and the next you're sounding as though you've swallowed a guppy.

Hiccups are nothing more than an annoying little spasm in the diaphragm, the thin, dome-like muscle that helps you breathe. Doctors suspect that hiccups are caused by a momentary irritation of the nerves that help control the diaphragm. Hiccups can occur at any time, but they're most common when your stomach is full or you've been drinking alcohol.

Hiccups aren't painful, but they can be embarrassing. To stop the "hics," here are some tips you may want to try.

Rub your palate. To stop hiccups, some doctors recommend gently massaging the palate (the roof of your mouth) with a cotton swab for several minutes. This may help calm the nervous reflexes that are causing the spasms.

Plug your ears. Some experts have found that plugging your ears with your fingers can help stop hiccups. This appears to stimulate the vagus nerve, which may play a role in causing the spasms.

Drink some water. No, you don't have to stand on your head at the same time. The act of swallowing helps interrupt the hiccup cycle, which sometimes stops it cold. Some people have found, in fact, that drinking from the side of the glass farthest away from you (the opposite side) is especially helpful.

Hold your breath. Taking a deep breath and holding it temporarily changes your body's balance of oxygen and carbon dioxide, which will sometimes stop the hiccups. Breathing into a paper bag for a minute may have the same effect.

Breathe deeply. Doing deep breathing exercises, in which you slowly draw a lot of air into your lungs and just as slowly let it out, can help calm your whole body, including the excitable diaphragm muscle that's causing the hiccups.

Massage your sides. According to acupressurists, there are two points just below your ribs straight down from the nipples that "control" abdominal activity. Pressing on these points for several minutes may interrupt the reflexes that are causing the hiccups.

HIVES

When we think of allergies we usually think of hay fever—the sneezing, runny nose, and itchy eyes that tell us spring has finally sprung. But there are many other kinds of allergies, as well, and it's not always the nose that's affected. For some people, coming into contact with the "wrong" things, like pollen, certain plants, or even ingredients in foods, can cause the skin to break out in ugly, itchy red blotches known as hives.

Hives occur when the body produces too much histamine, a natural chemical that's released when you're exposed to pollen or other allergens. Even if you don't have allergies you can still get hives—emotional stress and hot or cool weather can bring them on in some people.

The only way to prevent hives is to avoid whatever it is you're sensitive to. Since this isn't always possible, what you need are easy, practical solutions to relieve the discomfort. Here's what doctors recommend.

WHEN TO SEE THE DOCTOR

Most hives disappear on their own within a day or two, leaving no trace or scar. A problem that's similar to hives, however, is much more serious. If you have a condition called angioedema, which may be caused by an allergic reaction to foods (often to seafood or strawberries) or drugs, you may develop large welts beneath the skin that can cause intense swelling. You may have stomach cramps and diarrhea, as well. If you have any of these symptoms, or if the swelling is occurring near your throat or mouth or you're having trouble breathing, call your doctor right away.

Cool your skin. Research suggests that cooling your body will help shrink blood vessels, reducing the amount of histamine that reaches your skin. The next time you have hives, try taking cool showers or baths, or applying cool compresses. The less histamine reaches your skin, the quicker the hives will disappear.

Avoid the heat. Just as cold helps shrink the blood vessels, heating your body causes them to dilate, increasing the amount of histamine that reaches your skin. So when hives come out of hiding, it's a good idea to avoid hot showers and generally keep your body cool until the outbreak passes.

Think pink. Calamine lotion, available in pharmacies, is a time-proven remedy for hives. It won't make them go away, but it can be very helpful for easing the itch and irritation.

Reach for milk of magnesia. This traditional over-the-counter remedy is somewhat alkaline, which can be very effective for soothing hives. Pour some on a cotton ball and apply it to your skin several times a day. You should start feeling better right away.

Stop the histamine. Because the chemical histamine causes hives, doctors often recommend that people with hives take an antihistamine, such as Benadryl. These medications are safe and effective, and will often relieve the problem within a few days.

Look around you. You can get hives from so many different things, it's not always easy to figure out what's causing the problem. If you get hives often, it's worth taking the time to review *everything* you recently came into contact with—what you ate and drank, where you were, what you smelled. If you're able to figure out what's causing the problem, it will be a lot easier to prevent in the future.

HOT FLASHES

The word "menopause" comes from Greek words meaning "month" and "cessation." It refers to the time in a woman's life when the monthly menstrual cycle begins slowing down and finally stops entirely. Most women get through this stage without serious discomfort. But about 80 percent of women going through menopause will occasionally experience hot flashes. These are caused by declining estrogen levels, which make blood vessels in the skin periodically dilate. The rush of blood can result in sensations of searing heat, along with flushing and night sweats.

Hot flashes aren't dangerous, but they can be extremely uncomfortable. Here are some proven ways to turn down the heat.

WHEN TO SEE THE DOCTOR

Menopause isn't a disease and most women sail through this time in their lives without serious problems. But the declining levels of estrogen that accompany menopause may increase your risk for other, long-term problems, like osteoporosis or heart disease. To reduce these risks, doctors sometimes recommend that women be given supplemental doses of estrogen. Called hormone replacement therapy, this can help protect the bones and the heart, while at the same time reducing hot flashes and other uncomfortable symptoms of menopause. It's a good idea to see your doctor at the first signs of menopause to find out if this therapy is right for you.

Put tofu on the menu. Along with tempeh and other soy foods, tofu contains natural compounds called phytoestrogens, which are similar to the estrogen the body produces naturally. Research has shown that women who get a lot of soy foods in their diet are much less likely to have hot flashes.

Try an herbal cure. Natural practitioners often recommend that women having hot flashes take a Chinese herb called dong quai. Sold in tablet form in health food stores, dong quai may be very helpful for turning down the heat.

Take some vitamin E. Many physicians recommend that women having hot flashes take 400 IU of vitamin E twice a day, which can reduce their frequency and severity. Vitamin E can have side effects when taken in large doses, however, so check with your doctor before taking it.

94

Dress for the change. The body's thermostat is naturally set a little higher when you're going through menopause. It's important to do everything you can to keep cool. This includes dressing in layers (so you can take clothes off when you start feeling hot), wearing natural fabrics that "breathe," and keeping the temperature in the house a little lower.

Give up the cigarettes. Research has shown that some of the chemicals in tobacco smoke can cause estrogen levels to dip, making hot flashes even worse.

Help yourself relax. There's some evidence that hot flashes are caused in part by high levels of a chemical in the brain called norepinephrine. Reducing stress—by meditating, doing yoga, or deep breathing—can cause norepinephrine levels to fall, which may help reduce the frequency of hot flashes.

INSECT BITES AND STINGS

Mark Twain once said that God loved the fly, which is why He made so many of them. The same might be said of mosquitoes, spiders, bees, and the zillions of other biting, stinging creatures that seem to have nothing better to do than make your life miserable.

Insects were on earth long before we were and they'll be here long after we're gone. If you spend any time outdoors, there's simply no way to avoid them—or the painful, itchy consequences. But there are ways to get quick relief from close encounters with the buggy kind. Here's what doctors recommend you try.

WHEN TO SEE THE DOCTOR

Most people who have been bitten or stung by insects won't experience anything worse than a little itching and perhaps a painful welt. If you have allergies, however, insect bites and stings can be dangerous. In fact, about 100 people die in the United States each year from bee stings—that's 83 more than die from poisonous snake bites and grizzly bear attacks combined. If you've been stung by an insect and are dizzy, nauseated, or having trouble breathing, consider it an emergency. You could be having an allergic reaction called anaphylaxis, which can be life-threatening. You need to get to a doctor immediately.

Scrape off the stinger. When you've been stung by a bee, the stinger usually stays in the skin, where it keeps releasing venom. To reduce pain and prevent swelling, it's important to remove the stinger as soon as possible. Don't pull it out, because squeezing the stinger can cause it to release more venom into the skin. A better strategy is to scrape it out, using a credit card or stiff cardboard.

Paste on relief. Applying a paste made from baking soda and water directly to bites and stings can help draw out the venom, which will provide quick relief and prevent the pain from getting worse.

Get help from the kitchen. Another way to stop the pain of bites and stings is to apply a paste made from a meat tenderizer that contains papain. This substance helps break down the proteins in insect venom, reducing the pain-causing punch.

Cool the area. Covering insect bites and stings with a cool, damp cloth will help reduce swelling and provide instant pain relief. You also can put ice in a plastic bag and apply that instead.

Dress in muted colors. Insects are attracted to bright colors (which is why many flowers are adorned with brilliant reds and yellows). To stop insects from seeing *you* as their meal ticket, it's a good idea to wear subdued, dark-colored clothing when you're going to be spending time outdoors.

No scents makes good sense. Just as insects are attracted to bright colors, they're also attracted to sweet-smelling, flowery perfumes and soaps. When you're going camping, experts say, leave the scents behind, including scented deodorants.

Load up on garlic. It's not only vampires that are scared off by garlic. Some experts believe that eating garlic before going outside will make you less attractive to biting bugs.

Get plenty of thiamine. This vitamin, also called vitamin B1, may give your perspiration an odor that many insects find unappealing, although it's undetectable by humans.

INSOMNIA

We all battle sleeplessness once in awhile. Problems at work, a fight with your spouse, or simply a subtle shift in your body's "clock" will occasionally lead to sleepless nights. For some people, however, getting to sleep is an endless battle. Doctors estimate that forty to fifty million Americans, or half of all adults, will suffer from sleep problems. And when you get older, falling asleep may get even harder.

Everyone needs a different amount of sleep. Some people get five hours a night and wake up full of energy. Others are exhausted if they get less than nine or ten hours. What this means is that insomnia is a very personal thing. As a general rule, if you're suddenly getting less sleep than usual and are paying the price the next morning, you probably have insomnia and need to do something about it. Here's what doctors recommend.

Clear your head before you go to bed. Doctors estimate that about half of insomnia is caused by mental and emotional stress. This makes sense, as anyone who's tossed and turned the night before (or after) a stressful day can attest. You can't eliminate stress, but you can turn down the volume before you hit the hay. Sleep experts advise using the last half-hour of your day to wind down and clear your mind. Don't pore over your daily planner or scribble notes for tomorrow. Just relax. Spend a few minutes on the porch listening to the sounds of the night. Read for a bit, or give a little time to your hobby. Emptying the stress from your mind, even temporarily, will help prevent it from keeping you awake later on.

Pour a glass of milk. A glass of warm milk is a traditional remedy for sleepless nights, and now there's good evidence to show it works. Milk—along with turkey and cheese—contains an amino acid that's called tryptophan. The body converts tryptophan to serotonin—a natural chemical that helps the body regulate its sleep cycles. Having a little milk before bed—it can be warm or cold—will give your brain the message that it's time to be shutting down for the night.

98

Ask your doctor about melatonin. Another natural chemical that can help you sleep is called melatonin. Produced by the brain, melatonin helps set your internal clock, so your body knows when it's time to wake up and when to start getting sleepy. As you get older, the brain starts producing less melatonin—which is why doctors sometimes recommend that people with insomnia take melatonin supplements. Even small amounts—between one-half and one milligram—may help you sleep better. You can get melatonin at natural food stores, pharmacies, and even some grocery stores.

Pour a cup of herbal tea. Alternative practitioners believe that teas made from chamomile, valerian, or passion flower can be very helpful for calming you down and helping you get to sleep more quickly. Don't drink black tea at bedtime, however, because it contains caffeine.

Speaking of coffee, don't drink three cups after dinner and expect to sleep well that night. Caffeine is a powerful stimulant. Even when you're used to it, drinking coffee at night can lengthen the time it takes to fall asleep, and will also make the sleep you do get less restful.

Have a soothing soak. Few things are more relaxing than a long soak in a warm bath. Many people, in fact, start receiving overtures from the sandman even before they're out of the tub.

Make your days active. Research has shown that people who exercise during the day sleep a lot better than folks who are more sedentary. It's important, however, to get your exercise no later than the early evening. Exercise stimulates the brain and body, and doing it at night can make you too energized to fall asleep easily.

Say goodnight to nightcaps. Even though alcohol can help you fall asleep more quickly, it disturbs the overall quality of your sleep. That's why people who drink at night are often tired the next day, even when they got plenty of sleep.

99

JET LAG

Our bodies have internal clocks that are far more powerful than we realize. The time you wake up, when you eat, and when you bed down for the night are all determined by this internal clock.

Most of the time, your body's clock corresponds to your daily schedule—which is why you wake up at the start of the day and go to sleep at the end. When you travel across time zones, however, all of a sudden your body's clock and the "external" clocks are out of sync. When you fly from New York to Los Angeles, for example, the clock in your hotel may say it's 7 p.m., but your body thinks that it's 10 p.m. and time to go to sleep.

Jet lag can make you tired and forgetful. It throws off your sleep schedule, so you may have trouble falling asleep or wake up too early. In some cases, people with jet lag feel irritable, lose their appetites, or even have digestive problems such as heartburn or indigestion.

You don't have to stay home to beat jet lag. Making a few changes in your habits—before and after you travel—will help put things right. Here's how.

Stock up on sleep. You can't store sleep like pennies in a jar, but getting extra sleep before you travel can go a long way toward helping you feel refreshed when you arrive.

Plan time to unwind. Sleep experts recommend timing your travel so you arrive at your destination fairly early in the evening. This will give you time to have a good dinner and unwind before going to bed. Try to make yourself go to bed at the new time.

Of course, the rules are slightly different depending on the direction you're traveling. If you're flying east, it's going to be later when you arrive, so you may want to leave a little bit earlier in the day. Flying west, on the other hand, can cause you to lose a few hours, so you may want to book your flight a little bit later.

Stock up on fluids. Airline cabins are incredibly dry. Many people get dehydrated before they reach their destinations—and dehydration makes jet lag worse. Doctors recommend drinking a lot of water or juice before you leave home, as well as on the plane. Don't drink alcohol, however, because it can make dehydration worse.

Keep moving. It's not exactly easy to move around on the plane, but staying active will help you stay energized and refreshed. At the very least you should walk the aisles periodically and do simple stretching exercises in your seat. When you arrive at your destination, take a little time to walk around or, if your hotel has a pool or gym, get in some exercise.

Spend some time outdoors. Your body's internal clock is partially regulated by sunlight. Spending time outdoors when you arrive at your new destination will help your body clock adjust more quickly to the transition.

LACTOSE INTOLERANCE

Judging from the impressive lineup of milk mustaches in newspaper and magazine advertisements, you'd think that everyone is drinking milk. But the truth is, many adults can't stomach milk or other dairy foods.

Doctors estimate that up to 70 percent of the world's adult population and about thirty to fifty million Americans may have difficulty digesting lactose, a sugar found in milk, cheese, and other dairy foods. The reason for this is that adults often don't produce enough lactase, the enzyme needed to digest the lactose in dairy foods. When your body can't digest lactose, you may have gas, bloating, or diarrhea. Doctors call this problem lactose intolerance.

Some people are born with lactose intolerance. More often, the problem gradually gets worse with age, which is why children can usually drink milk while many adults can't. Both men and women can develop lactose intolerance, but it's more urgent a problem for women. Why? It makes it harder for them to get the calcium they need to prevent osteoporosis, a bone-thinning disease that mainly strikes women.

If you have lactose intolerance, even small amounts of dairy foods may make you quite ill. Most people, however, can enjoy some dairy foods without having problems. In addition, there are a number of ways to get the benefits of dairy without the problems. Here's how.

Start small. Evidence suggests that most people with lactose intolerance are able to enjoy small amounts of dairy foods. Try having a small glass of milk and seeing if it agrees with you. Then gradually increase the amount until you discover your upper limit. In most cases, people with lactose intolerance will tolerate dairy foods better when they have them with meals.

Have a little yogurt. To get the benefits of dairy without the problems, many people turn to yogurt. Yogurt that contains live cultures of bacteria is easier for the body to digest than milk or other dairy foods. In fact, eating yogurt will often make it easier for you to digest other dairy foods, as well. Frozen yogurt doesn't work, however, because freezing deactivates the live cultures.

Take supplemental protection. To replace the lactase your body isn't producing naturally, you can buy lactase supplements in pharmacies and some grocery stores. These supplements may be taken in pill or capsule form, or simply as drops that you put in a glass of milk. Or you can buy reduced-lactose milk, which has far less lactose than regular milk.

Explore milk substitutes. Even if you can't drink cow's milk, you can enjoy other forms of milk, such as soy milk. Many people with lactose intolerance find that buttermilk is much easier to digest than regular milk.

Or try it with chocolate. Evidence suggests that adding a little cocoa to milk makes it easier for the body to digest. To get the benefits of calcium with a little chocolate flavor, it's certainly worth a try.

Buy hard cheeses. Different cheeses contain different amounts of lactose. The hard cheeses, like Swiss or extra-sharp cheddar, are among the easiest for people who have lactose intolerance to digest.

103

Concentrate on calcium. The worst part about having lactose intolerance is that it's often hard to get all the calcium you need without drinking milk or eating cheese. To make up for this missing mineral, it's a good idea to eat calcium-rich foods like broccoli, kidney beans, collard greens, tofu, and dark green, leafy vegetables. In addition, orange juice is often fortified with calcium.

WHEN TO SEE THE DOCTOR

Many people with lactose intolerance are able to diagnose the problem themselves by giving up dairy foods for a while, then having a glass of milk and seeing what happens. If you suspect you have lactose intolerance, but you aren't sure, call your doctor. He can perform a test that will measure how effectively your body breaks down lactose.

LARYNGITIS

It's not a serious problem, but it *sounds* awful. When you get laryngitis, which can be caused by a cold, the flu, or simply using your voice too much, you can start sounding like Marlon Brando in the *Godfather*. Some people lose their voices entirely for a few days or even longer.

WHEN TO SEE THE DOCTOR

Laryngitis rarely causes anything worse than a little hoarseness and a tickly throat. If the pain is severe, however, or if you're wheezing or coughing up blood, you need to see your doctor immediately. In some cases the upper airways will get so swollen that it's hard for air to get through. Without treatment, the airways could close entirely. So it's important to get medical help right away.

When laryngitis is stealing your voice, fight back with these easy tips.

Sip warm tea with lemon. This traditional remedy is often used by professional singers whose voices are about to give out. Tea contains tannic acids, which can help soothe inflamed tissues in the throat. Adding lemon to the tea will help cut through mucus, which will also help bring your voice back to normal.

Pour down the water. Drinking eight to twelve glasses of water a day will help lubricate the larynx, which is essential for stopping laryngitis. It's best to drink water that's room temperature. Water that's too hot or too cold can irritate the larynx even more.

Settle in for a hot shower. Breathing hot, steamy air will help relax your throat and airways so you can breathe—and talk—more easily. Using a humidifier at night can also be very helpful.

Forget the salt water. This is one traditional remedy to skip when you have laryngitis. Gargling with salt water can dry out the throat even more. In addition, the vibrations of gargling cause the vocal cords to slap together, which can increase the irritation.

Don't take aspirin. Even though aspirin can help relieve the discomfort of a sore throat and laryngitis, it also slows the time it takes your body to form blood clots. Since laryngitis may be caused by minor injuries to the vocal cords, taking aspirin can actually slow the healing time.

Handle your voice with care. If you've been spending weekends cheering your daughter's softball team, your vocal cords may pay the price. When you have laryngitis, it's essential to speak quietly for awhile—or, whenever possible, not at all. And forget about whispering: It's even harder on your vocal cords than talking in a normal voice.

MENSTRUAL CRAMPS

Nearly every woman will have menstrual cramps at some time in her life. But for some women, the cramps are severe not just occasionally, but month after month. Doctors call this condition dysmenorrhea. It literally means "difficult monthly flow," and that's an understatement. In many cases, the cramps are accompanied by other problems, such as nausea, diarrhea, or overall achiness.

It's unfortunate, but cramps are a normal part of menstruation. But that doesn't mean you can't get relief. There are a number of strategies that will help reduce monthly pain. Here are a few you may want to try.

WHEN TO SEE THE DOCTOR

Mild menstrual cramps are normal, but they shouldn't be agonizing. If you're experiencing a lot of pain or other symptoms, or if your menstrual periods are getting less regular or you're bleeding heavily, it's important to see your doctor. Cramps can be a symptom of a number of underlying problems, including endometriosis, pelvic inflammatory disease, or even cysts or tumors. Your doctor will want to do a pelvic exam, and possibly blood and urine tests, to make sure nothing serious is going on. In addition, she may give you prescription drugs that will help relieve the pain.

Try some soothing heat. Putting a hot water bottle or a heating pad on your abdomen will help ease the discomfort of cramps. As long as you keep the temperature at safe levels, you can leave the heat in place for about twenty minutes at a time, and repeat it every few hours throughout the day. Taking a hot shower or a long bath can also be very soothing, doctors say. A little pampering can do wonders.

Put your trust in medications. For most women, over-the-counter pain pills such as aspirin and ibuprofen are very effective at stopping cramps. These drugs block the effects of chemicals in the body called prostaglandins, which are responsible for causing much of the pain. You can take these drugs when cramps begin, but they're more effective if you start taking them a day or two ahead of time and continue taking them until the cramps go away.

Take a long walk. Doctors aren't sure why, but evidence suggests that walking, swimming, or other forms of exercise will help make cramps less troublesome.

Stretch for relief. For quick relief from cramps, try this stretch: Get on your knees, then sit back so your bottom rests on your heels. Bend forward until your chest is resting on your thighs and your forehead is touching the floor. Hold the stretch for a minute or two. Many women swear that it's the best and quickest way to quiet cramps.

Give up coffee for a few days. For some women, giving up caffeine—which is found not only in coffee, but also in chocolate, cola, and some teas—helps make menstrual cramps less severe. You don't have to give up caffeine entirely—just for a few days until the cramping subsides.

Get plenty of minerals. Doctors have found that getting enough calcium, which is found mainly in dairy foods, and magnesium, found in beans, whole-grains, and a variety of vegetables, can be very helpful for reducing cramping.

MIGRAINES

Migraine headaches can be ferociously painful. People who get migraines simply cannot function during an attack. They lose days from work and often get physically ill. It's not uncommon during an attack for people to lock themselves in a dark room, hoping against hope that the pain will go away.

All migraines cause pain, but different varieties cause other symptoms, as well. Classic migraines, for example, may cause auras—strange visual changes that can make you see sparkling or flashing lights or zigzag lines. People with classic migraines may develop blind spots and are often intensely sensitive to light. The aura usually begins about half an hour before the pain sets in, then it disappears.

Unlike classic migraines, common migraines don't cause auras. Instead, people with common migraines may experience emotional changes including depression before attacks. A third type of migraine, called the complicated migraine, is a combination of classic and common migraines. People with complicated migraines will have auras before the pain, which don't always go away once the headache begins. In fact, the auras may last longer than the pain itself.

Doctors still aren't sure what causes migraines. They appear to be related to the alternating expansion and contraction of blood vessels in the brain. Women are three times as likely as men to get migraines, and there appears to be a hereditary link. And for some reason, migraines rarely occur during pregnancy.

Migraines can be extremely serious and doctors usually treat them with powerful prescription drugs. But there are also things you can do at home to blunt the pain and possibly help prevent them from coming back.

WHEN TO SEE THE DOCTOR

There's nothing simple about migraines. They're hard to treat, hard to prevent, and tend to recur. Most people with migraines learn the best tricks for handling them at home—turning out the lights, for example, or just taking it easy for a day. But if the headaches are accompanied by seizures or severe confusion, or if the pain is significantly different or more severe than usual, you should call your doctor right away.

Cool it down. At the first sign of an attack, splash your face with cold water, then apply an ice pack wrapped in towels to your head and lie down in a dark, quiet room. The ice will constrict blood vessels, which can reduce irritation of nerves in the head.

Head for bed. Doctors agree that sleep is one of the best ways of stopping a migraine. It's not always easy to sleep when you're in pain, of course, but it's worth giving it a try. Turn out the lights, breathe slowly and deeply, and do everything possible to relax. If you're able to sleep, there's a good chance you'll wake up pain-free.

Relax often. Prevention may be your best bet when it comes to migraines. Research suggests that reducing stress and relaxing will help reduce the risk of migraines. This only works if you do it regularly, however. In fact, people who don't relax very often are more likely to get migraines during vacations or on weekends than at other times— probably because the body has become so accustomed to an adrenaline-fueled lifestyle that it's unable to adapt to the change. It's essential to make rest and relaxation a regular part of your schedule, doctors say.

109

Watch what you eat. Certain foods are notorious migraine triggers. The worst offenders include red wine, chocolate, aged cheese, milk, chicken livers, meats preserved with nitrates (like bacon, hot dogs, and deli meats), and anything prepared with monosodium glutamate (MSG).

Have a handful of nuts. Researchers have found that people prone to migraines often get too little magnesium in their diets. Along with dark green, leafy vegetables and fruits, nuts are an excellent source of this important mineral, which has been shown to help relax the muscles throughout the body, including in the head and scalp. Other good magnesium sources are brown rice, spinach, haddock, oatmeal, potatoes, bananas, beans, and yogurt.

Stay in shape. Doctors have found that people who stay in shape are less likely to have migraines than those who are more sedentary—probably because people who exercise tend to have less stress as well as better circulation and stronger blood vessels. It's a good idea to get some aerobic exercise—by walking, jogging, swimming, biking, or even dancing—three or four times a week.

Although exercise can help prevent migraines, it's not a treatment. Moving around when you're in the midst of an attack will make you feel worse instead of better.

MORNING SICKNESS

If you've never had a baby before, the first few months of pregnancy can definitely take some getting used to. The problem isn't weight gain or food cravings. The real problem is trying to get through an entire day without dashing for the bathroom. It's called "morning sickness," but your stomach doesn't wear a watch. Morning, noon, or night— you can never be sure when your stomach is going to start feeling queasy.

Doctors aren't sure what causes morning sickness or why it affects some women and not others, or some pregnancies and not others. Here's what they do know. Morning sickness usually occurs between the sixth and thirteenth week of pregnancy, and generally starts to settle down after that. It's thought that changing levels of hormones or blood sugars are probably responsible.

Morning sickness isn't dangerous and it isn't uncommon (as though that makes you feel any better). But it can be dreadfully uncomfortable. Here are a few ways to keep your stomach calm.

WHEN TO SEE THE DOCTOR

Morning sickness can make you feel miserable, but it's a normal part of pregnancy. The exception is if you're also losing weight or you can't eat anything all day long. When morning sickness is this severe, for your sake and the baby's you need to call your doctor immediately.

Keep crackers at your bedside. One of the best foods for beating morning sickness is unsalted crackers. Doctors often recommend that women who are expecting morning

111

sickness eat crackers first thing in the morning and as often during the day as they wish. Putting food in your stomach will help keep it calm. Crackers are easy for the body to digest, making them the perfect "queasy food." You may even want to keep the crackers right by your bedside to eat the minute you wake up; otherwise, by the time you get up and get dressed it might be too late.

Pour a little ginger. Ginger has been used for centuries for easing a variety of stomach troubles, and many doctors feel it's an effective remedy for morning sickness, as well. You can buy ginger tea at health food stores. Or take ginger supplements, which appear to work just as well. (For more on using ginger, see the Nausea chapter on page 118.)

Eat early and often. When your stomach is on edge, you don't want to overburden it by eating too much all at once. Most women find that eating several small meals a day is more comfortable than having a few large ones.

Drink plenty of fluids. When you've been vomiting because of morning sickness, your body loses valuable fluids—and dehydration will make your stomach even more unsteady. It's a good idea to drink as much water as you comfortably can—at least eight to twelve glasses a day, doctors say. If you'd like something with a little taste, juices and sports drinks also are good.

Have a frozen treat. Many women find that frozen-fruit bars, the ones made with real juice, can hit the spot when nothing else wants to stay down. They're slightly sweet, so they help replace sugars you may be losing if you're vomiting. They're also filled with water, so they can help satisfy your daily fluid needs.

Let your stomach be your guide. There are no hard and fast rules for choosing "comfort" foods. Some women do best with bland foods like rice and crackers, while others may prefer salads, beans, or fresh vegetables. You'll just have to experiment a bit to see which foods cause the least problems—and which you'll want to avoid. As a rule, doctors say, you should plan on avoiding fried or very strong-flavored foods, since they're often hard to digest and are more likely to trigger morning sickness.

Get some fresh air. When you've been in a stuffy room and your stomach won't hold still, getting a breath of fresh air can help calm things down. Just opening the window can help settle your stomach. Better yet, take a walk. Many doctors recommend mild exercise for all pregnant women, especially those with morning sickness.

MOTION SICKNESS

There's a lot to be said for the good old days when people got around mainly by foot power. Cars, boats, and airplanes may get us there faster, but our stomachs don't always appreciate the difference. Nearly everyone has motion sickness from time to time, and some folks can't even ride across town without sitting by an open window.

Motion sickness is essentially caused by breakdowns in communication. Your eyes are telling your body that you're barely moving, while your other senses know very well that you're rocking along. The brain doesn't like the confusion, and it responds by sending nausea signals.

If you're prone to motion sickness, you'll never stop it entirely—you certainly won't be first in line to try the new roller coaster at the amusement park. But doctors have found a few ways to help your various senses work together and also to keep the stomach calm. Here is what some doctors advise.

Stay active. If you've ever taken a long road trip you know it's the passengers and not the driver who get car sick. Researchers have found that keeping your brain busy is one of the best ways to stop the queasies. An obvious solution, of course, is to put yourself in the driver's seat. Or think of ways to keep your mind active. Some people play mental games, while others count license plates. The busier you are, the more stable your stomach will be.

Sit up front. Researchers have found that passengers who sit in the front seat of a car usually have less nausea than those in the back—probably because when you're sitting up front it's easier to see the car's motion, which helps keep the other senses from sending contradictory— "We're moving! No, we're not!"—signals to the brain.

Scan the horizon. Wherever you're sitting, it's a good idea to let your eyes scan the horizon. Giving your brain the big-picture view can help keep nausea at bay.

Settle your stomach with ginger. Long used by sailors to keep their stomachs calm, ginger has been shown to be as effective at stopping nausea as some over-the-counter drugs. Ginger tea is effective, although many experts recommend taking ginger supplements, which you can get from health food stores. Take a few capsules before leaving and continue taking them as you travel, following the directions on the label.

114

Put something in your stomach. Researchers have found that an empty stomach becomes very irritable and unstable and much more prone to nausea. Before getting in the car or on the boat, stop and eat something first. You're better off eating easy-to-digest carbohydrates, such as rice and potatoes, than high-fat foods, which are hard to digest.

Press for relief. Some experts believe that putting pressure on a certain point on the wrist, called an acupressure point, will help stop motion sickness. The point is located in the middle of your wrist, palm-side up, about one inch above the crease. When your stomach starts acting up, exert gentle pressure for as long as it takes to get relief. You can even buy elastic wrist bands (called SeaBands) that automatically press on this point. The bands are often sold in boating supply stores.

Close the book. Some people are lucky enough to be able to read when they're in motion, but most folks who are prone to motion sickness find it's about the worst thing to do. Your eyes see the book and send a message you're sitting still, but the other senses know otherwise—and this can lead to motion sickness.

MUSCLE PAIN

We usually don't give a lot of thought to our muscles. As long as we can do the basics—hoisting a child, hauling out the garbage, or carrying a box of books upstairs—we take them for granted. Then one day we push them a little harder than usual and spend the next few days limping about. At that point it's hard to think about anything else.

Your body has more than 650 muscles, from the tiny muscles in the face to the enormously strong muscles in the thighs. Your body's muscles account for about half your body weight and they consume roughly one-fourth of the total calories you take in. Even when you're sleeping, the muscles do a lot of work. If they're not exercised regularly or if you push them too hard, they're likely to get hurt.

Aching muscles usually recover quite quickly—if you take fast action. Here are a few things you'll want to try.

Put the pain on ice. The most powerful remedy for muscle aches is applying cold, which constricts blood vessels and slows the flow of blood, preventing swelling. If the muscle ache is in your arm or leg, you may be able to ice it down simply by putting some cubes in a plastic bag and holding them in place for fifteen or twenty minutes. If your whole body is aching, you may want to fill the bath with cool water and settle in for awhile.

Try hot and cold. Some athletic trainers recommend that people with muscle aches start out by taking a hot shower, followed by a cold-water spritz. Repeating this cycle several times can cause the blood vessels to alternately open wide and snap shut, which will help flush pain-causing lactic acid (a by-product of muscle metabolism) from the muscles.

Wrap it up. For worse-than-average muscle pain, doctors recommend compressing the muscle by wrapping it with a gauze strip or a special compress bandage. Putting gentle pressure on a muscle will help prevent swelling and inflammation. Don't wrap the bandage too tightly, however; it could cut off circulation.

Raise it high. Another way to help prevent swelling and ease the pain is to elevate the sore muscle above the level of your heart.

Take advantage of aspirin. This tried-and-true pain remedy works as well for muscle aches as for other kinds of pain. Ibuprofen also is effective. Although acetaminophen will help ease pain, it has little effect against inflammation. Pain reliever labels should indicate which are effective in relieving muscle pain.

Put your hands to work. Rubbing a muscle is one of the best ways to ease the aches and pains. Massage—whether you're doing it to yourself or it's being done to you—improves the flow of blood and other fluids through the area, and also helps carry away muscle waste products that cause pain. It's safe to massage most muscle injuries, but you may find that it's simply too painful. If that's the case, don't bother—it may do more harm than good.

Take time to warm up. The best way to prevent muscle pain is to take a few minutes to warm up before doing any strenuous physical activity. You don't have to do anything fancy. Just jogging in place for a few minutes or stretching your legs, back, shoulders, and chest will help keep the muscles loose and limber so they're less likely to get hurt.

Get your vitamins. Research suggests that getting plenty of antioxidant vitamins—especially vitamins C and E—in your diet can help prevent muscle injuries. These vitamins are effective because they help block the effects of harmful oxygen molecules in the body called free radicals, which otherwise can contribute to tissue damage and pain. The best sources for vitamin C include fresh fruits and vegetables. Vitamin E is only found in a few foods, like nuts and cooking oils, which is why many doctors recommend taking vitamin E supplements.

Pour a sports drink. "Athletic" drinks such as Gatorade are high in carbohydrates and electrolytes, and some experts believe that drinking them when you're physically active can help prevent muscle soreness later on.

117

NAUSEA

Everyone's stomach does gymnastics once in a while. Sometimes it's because of something you ate, or the sight of blood, or because your stomach's a landlubber even though your heart's into sailing. And sometimes the stomach gets upset for no apparent reason at all.

Nausea usually isn't serious and will go away on its own fairly quickly. Here are a few tips for speeding it on its way.

WHEN TO SEE THE DOCTOR

Even though your stomach is surprisingly durable and does a hard day's work every day, it's also sensitive to changes throughout your body. When you're getting nauseated frequently and you don't know why, there could be an underlying problem and you should see your doctor.

Give ginger a try. People have been taking ginger for stomach troubles for thousands of years, and modern research suggests it works. When your stomach is turning upside down, you can soothe it fast by drinking a little ginger tea. Or take ginger supplements, which are just as effective.

Have a little cola. Doctors aren't sure why it works, but cola syrup, which you can get from some pharmacies, appears to keep stomachs calm. Ginger ale is also effective, although it's best not to drink it straight out of the can. Pour a glass and let it go flat. Then drink it down, doctors advise.

Brew some chamomile tea. Herbalists often recommend chamomile tea for soothing an upset stomach. You can buy chamomile at most grocery or natural food stores.

Give your stomach a break. When you're seeing green

118

and your stomach is doing its upside-down thing, you don't want to be eating a lot of rich, hard-to-digest foods. Instead, keep your diet simple. Doctors recommend eating "clear" foods, like broth or Jell-O, or easy-to-digest carbohydrates like potatoes, rice, or toast.

Take some B vitamins. Your body uses B vitamins to help metabolize proteins and fats. When you're feeling nauseated, taking a B-complex multivitamin may help you feel a little bit better.

Put acupressure to work. Oriental doctors believe that pressing on certain parts of the body can help stop nausea fast. They recommend pressing on the inside of your wrist, about an inch above the crease where it joins your hand. Maintain the pressure for about fifteen seconds, and repeat as often as necessary.

Practice mind over motion. Some people are able to beat nausea by deliberately taking their minds as far away from their upset tummies as possible. The next time you're feeling sick, shut your eyes and imagine a peaceful, soothing scene. It could be a beautiful sunset or sunny spot in the garden. Give yourself time to really focus on the scene— imagine how it looks, feels, and sounds. The more detail you're able to imagine, the less nausea you're going to have.

Hold still. Researchers have found that moving around can disturb the balance mechanism in the inner ear, which makes nausea worse. To keep your stomach calm, it's a good idea to sit or stand upright, and to move your head as little as possible.

NOSEBLEEDS

You don't have to square off with Mike Tyson to suffer a nosebleed. The membranes in the nose are very thin, with a delicate network of blood vessels very near the surface. Dry air, allergies, or even blowing your nose too hard can irritate the lining in the nose, causing nosebleeds.

Because the nose contains so many blood vessels, it can bleed a lot in a hurry. But it usually looks a lot worse than it really is. That's a small comfort, however, when it's your nose that's doing the bleeding. To stop nosebleeds fast, here's what doctors advise.

WHEN TO SEE THE DOCTOR

If you're getting frequent nosebleeds, call your doctor. There are a number of problems, including high blood pressure and infections, that can make the nose bleed very easily, so it's important to get it checked out.

Give it a pinch. The quickest way to stop a nosebleed is to sit on a chair or on the edge of your bed and firmly pinch your nose closed. Hold it closed for five to ten minutes. By stopping the flow of blood, you'll give it time to clot, which usually happens in a few minutes. Don't pack your nose with gauze or cotton, because it could pull off the clot when you remove it. And of course, don't blow your nose for a while, which could start the bleeding again.

Incidentally, it's important to lean forward or tilt your head to the side when trying to stop your nosebleed. Tilting your head backward will cause blood to drip down the back of your throat, which could make you nauseated.

Stop it at the source. If your nose keeps bleeding, try rolling some gauze into a tight cylinder and placing it under your upper lip. There are several blood vessels in this area, and the cylinder of gauze will help press them closed, so there's less blood flowing into the nose.

Put ice to work. Cold temperatures cause blood vessels to constrict, reducing the flow of blood. If your nose does not cease bleeding on its own, put some ice in a plastic bag, wrap it in a towel, and drape it over the bridge of your nose. In most cases the bleeding will stop within a few minutes.

Put more moisture in the air. Nosebleeds are often caused by dry air, especially in the winter. If you get nosebleeds often, your doctor may recommend plugging in a humidifier, which will make the air moister and easier on the lining of your nose. If you don't have a humidifier, here's another tip you may want to try: Fill several bowls with water and place them in different rooms in the house. The water will naturally evaporate and release water droplets into the air. If you have a green thumb, you may want to buy several houseplants, which will also help you keep the air moist.

Re-hydrate yourself. If you're not taking in enough fluids, tissues throughout your body, including in the nose, will get dry and irritated. Drinking a lot of water—eight to twelve glasses a day—will help keep your mucus membranes moist and protected.

Sniff some water. A quick way to lubricate the inside of the nose is simply to sniff some water. You can buy saline nose sprays at the pharmacy. Or simply mix a pinch of salt in a glass of lukewarm water and sniff it out of the palm of your hand. Then blow gently in a tissue to rid your nose of excess water.

Apply some protection. Many people treat a dry nose by rubbing on a little petroleum jelly. Or you can apply a thin layer of gel from an aloe vera leaf. Aloe is very soothing and may help your nose heal more quickly.

Eat well. Research has shown that a diet rich in vitamins C and E, as well as the B vitamins, can help strengthen blood vessels and prevent bleeding. Vitamin E is especially good because it's a natural anti-inflammatory that will help stop swelling.

The best way to get plenty of these vitamins is to eat a well-balanced diet with plenty of fruits, vegetables, whole grains, and legumes. In addition, you may want to take a vitamin E supplement because this nutrient is hard to get from foods alone.

Put out the smokes—and drink less, too. Cigarette smoke is extremely drying and can damage the delicate blood vessels inside the nose. Alcohol also dries the nose because it's a diuretic, meaning it removes more moisture from the body than the drink puts back in.

OSTEOPOROSIS

We think of bones as being hard and durable—so durable, in fact, that we often forget they're living tissue. But bones, like tissues throughout your body, are constantly breaking down. Your body needs lots of calcium, and your bones are the main storehouse. When calcium levels in the body dip, calcium is removed from the bones and then it is transported through the bloodstream. Over time, your bones reabsorb calcium from the blood and "redeposit" it, which keeps them strong.

As a woman ages and begins edging toward menopause, however, she produces less estrogen, the hormone that helps control the rate at which calcium is reabsorbed into the bones. As estrogen levels fall, the bones may begin giving up more calcium than they take in. As a result, they get softer, weaker, and more prone to fractures. Doctors call this condition osteoporosis. Men also get osteoporosis, but much less often than women do.

Doctors estimate that approxmately twenty-four million Americans have osteoporosis. It's responsible for about a third of all hip and vertebral fractures in people fifty years and older. It also causes back pain and, in some cases, a stooped posture as bones in the spine weaken and collapse.

Once you have osteoporosis, it can be very difficult to reverse the problems. But it's very easy to prevent, mainly by making simple changes in your diet and lifestyle. Here's what experts advise.

WHEN TO SEE THE DOCTOR

Osteoporosis is a very serious condition that should always be under a physician's care. Women going through menopause are especially at risk of developing osteoporosis. Other things that can increase your risk include surgery to remove the ovaries, smoking, heavy drinking, not getting enough calcium, or taking medications such as steroids. If you have any of these risk factors and haven't been checked for osteoporosis, it's probably time to make an appointment just to be safe.

Concentrate on calcium. By far the most important thing you can do to prevent and treat osteoporosis is to get more calcium. All women should get at least 1,000 milligrams of calcium a day. Women who are past menopause need even more, about 1,500 milligrams of calcium a day. Most women don't get anywhere near those amounts, and that's unfortunate because it's very easy to get all the calcium you need in your diet.

Dairy foods are the best sources of calcium. A cup of skim milk, for example, has over 300 milligrams of calcium. A cup of yogurt has a lot more, about 450 milligrams. Cheese is also good. A serving of mozzarella cheese, for example, has over 180 milligrams of calcium.

Even if you're not a big fan of dairy foods, there are plenty of other places to get calcium. Fortified orange juice, for example, contains about as much calcium as an equal serving of milk. You can also get a lot of calcium in leafy green vegetables, such as bok choy, kale, and broccoli.

Ask your doctor about supplements. If you're not getting enough calcium in your diet, your doctor may recommend that you take calcium supplements, which will easily provide all you need.

Don't forget the D. Your body needs vitamin D in order to absorb calcium. This is perhaps the easiest nutrient to get. All you have to do is spend a little time outdoors. Vitamin D is called the "sunshine vitamin" because your body produces it naturally whenever sunshine touches your skin. You can also get vitamin D by drinking fortified milk.

Consider hormone replacement. It's not for everyone, but some women past menopause will benefit from taking supplemental estrogen. Increasing the amount of estrogen in your body will vastly improve the bones' ability to absorb more calcium.

124

Cut back on colas. Colas and other soft drinks contain a substance called phosphoric acid, which can speed the removal of calcium from your bones.

Exercise regularly. Doctors at one time were nervous about recommending exercise to post-menopausal women because it was thought that vigorous activity might increase the risk of fractures in already weak bones. Experts now know, however, that regular exercise—especially weight-bearing exercise, such as walking and lifting weights—can actually cause the bones to take in more calcium, making them thicker and stronger. Swimming is great exercise because it puts virtually no stress on already weakened bones.

POISON IVY AND OAK

Mother Nature isn't always kind. Even though her gardens are a wonder to behold, they can contain a few unpleasant surprises. Not everyone is sensitive to poison oak or ivy, but if you are, their pointed, shiny leaves can give you a painful, itchy rash you won't soon forget.

Poison oak and ivy contain an oily resin called urushiol, which sticks to your skin at the slightest touch. You don't even have to touch a plant to get the rash. If your dog has been running in the woods, or you've been cutting weeds at the back of your yard, the oil can be passed from your dog's coat or the hoe's handle to you. What's more, it's incredibly potent. Experts have found that urushiol can stay active for years. This means you can get a rash from touching a tool handle that touched one of the poison plants last year or the year before that.

125

The best offense is a good defense. To avoid poison oak or poison ivy, you have to know what they look like. Poison ivy usually appears as low-growing patches, bushes, or creeping vines. The leaves are smooth-edged and glossy, radiating out from the stem in groups of three. Poison oak also grows as a bush or in patches. The leaves, too, are light to dark green and glossy. The edges aren't smooth, however, but jagged, and resemble oak leaves. When you're not sure if what you're looking at is poison oak or poison ivy, remember the hiker's adage: "Leaves of three? Let it be!"

If one of these plants has already put the bite on you, you have to act quickly to remove the oil before it triggers a rash. Here's how.

Scrub it off. Doctors have found that if you wash off all traces of the oil within ten minutes, you may be able to prevent the rash entirely or at least lessen its severity. Just rinsing with water won't help. You need to lather the area thoroughly with soap or a dish detergent, which will help break down the oil and remove it from your skin.

Milk does the body good. If the rash has already started, applying a milk compress can be very soothing. Soak gauze pads in milk and apply them to the rash. The milk will help dry the rash and also relieve the itching.

Reach for the oatmeal. One of the best ways to relieve a rash caused by poison oak or poison ivy is to fill the bath with lukewarm water and sprinkle in a little colloidal oatmeal, like Aveeno. This "softens" the water, which will soothe the rash and help it dry.

Freeze that itchy feeling. Applying an ice cube to the rash will quickly calm the itch and ease your discomfort. If the rash covers a large area, put some ice cubes in a plastic bag, wrap that in a towel, and lay it on the area for fifteen or twenty minutes.

Pick up some calamine lotion. This traditional favorite with the shocking pink color can quickly ease the rash caused by poison oak and ivy. Apply with a cotton ball.

POSTNASAL DRIP

You're usually not aware of it, but mucus from the sinuses is constantly sliding down the back of your throat. In fact, your body produces—and eliminates—about a cup of mucus a day. It's your body's way of keeping the nose and sinuses free of debris.

When you have a cold or allergies, however, your body can produce enormous amounts of mucus. What was a trickle can suddenly become a flood. So you clear your throat, cough a few times, then clear your throat again—and you still can't get rid of all that extra mucus. Postnasal drip isn't serious, but it can be maddeningly uncomfortable. How can you get rid of it?

Pour down the water. It won't prevent your body from producing mucus, but drinking lots of water will help thin the mucus and flush it from your throat before it starts getting irritating.

Snort some salt water. A quick way to clear out some of the mucus is to mix a quarter-teaspoon of table salt in a cup of water and snort some of the mixture into your nose, one nostril at a time. Then blow your nose, and finish up by gargling with the remainder of the saltwater mixture. This will help flush the mucus away.

Heat up the menu. Studies have shown that eating steamy or spicy foods will help thin the mucus so it flows more easily. In fact, just breathing the steam from a cup of hot soup will clear your head so you can breathe.

Keep your head up. Postnasal drip tends to be worse at night, when the position of your head causes mucus to slide down the back of your throat. Many people get relief by propping up the torso with pillows, which prevents the mucus from pooling at the back of the throat. Or you can raise the entire head of your bed by slipping bricks or pieces of wood under the legs.

WHEN TO SEE THE DOCTOR

If your postnasal drip is accompanied by pain and swelling in the "T" zone of your face or by a fever, you may have a sinus condition that requires a doctor's care.

PREMENSTRUAL DISCOMFORT

It begins at puberty and, for some women, doesn't end until menopause—thirty-five or forty years of cramping, bloating, mood swings, and other uncomfortable symptoms that may occur *every month*. It's called premenstrual discomfort, and doctors estimate that it affects as many as three out of four women at some time in their lives.

Premenstrual discomfort isn't a disease, even though it often feels like one. Caused mainly by complex changes in a woman's hormones prior to menstruation, premenstrual discomfort is usually most severe in women in their twenties and thirties, and it gradually gets less bothersome as the years go by.

It's a complex problem, with more than 150 different kinds of symptoms. Every woman experiences premenstrual discomfort differently. Until you reach menopause, you can't stop premenstrual discomfort entirely. But there are ways to make it a little more bearable. Here's what doctors advise.

Fill up on carbohydrates. Many women have food cravings in the days (or weeks) before their periods. Rather than giving in to the lure of sweets and high-fat fast foods, doctors recommend that you eat complex carbohydrates, like pasta and potatoes. These foods will provide quick, long-lasting energy. Plus, they're high in fiber, which has been shown to remove excess estrogen from the body. This is important because high levels of estrogen can increase premenstrual discomfort.

Get more B vitamins. Evidence suggests that eating foods that are high in B vitamins can help reduce mood swings, bloating, and other kinds of premenstrual discomfort. You can get a lot of B vitamins in chicken, turkey, and some kinds of fish. Bananas are also a rich source of B vitamins.

Cut back on salt. Whether you're sprinkling it on at the table or getting it in canned or take-out foods, salt causes the body to retain fluids, increasing the bloating that often precedes menstruation.

Drink a little less coffee. It's not a problem for everyone, but some women are sensitive to the caffeine in coffee, colas, and chocolate, which can result in mood swings as well as breast tenderness.

129

Try to keep moving. Any kind of exercise, even if it's just walking ten minutes a day, will help combat premenstrual discomfort. Exercise improves your body's circulation and helps keep hormone levels more stable. Some women have found, in fact, that even moderate exercise can relieve bloating and cramps almost immediately.

Heat away cramps. Most women will experience painful menstrual cramps from time to time. Putting a heating pad or a hot water bottle on your abdomen will increase blood flow to the area and help relieve the discomfort. Taking a hot bath or shower can also be very soothing.

Drink more water. It sounds odd, but drinking more water can actually relieve bloating because drinking stimulates your body to urinate more frequently.

WHEN TO SEE THE DOCTOR

The problem with premenstrual discomfort is that almost all of the symptoms can be caused by other, more serious conditions. If your symptoms always appear before your period and disappear soon after it begins, there isn't likely to be a problem. If the discomfort doesn't go away, however, or if it gradually gets worse over time, you need to see your doctor for a checkup.

PSORIASIS

Your skin is completely waterproof; it protects your insides, and it's self-repairing. Forget nylon, rayon, and other "miracle" fabrics—your skin puts them all to shame.

We think of the skin as being invariable, but in fact it's changing all the time. Every day individual skin cells grow, die, fall off, and then are replaced by new cells. This process generally lasts about four weeks. When you have psoriasis, however, the entire process is accelerated. Skin cells go through their life cycles in four days instead of a month. The cells aren't formed quite right, so they don't shed as quickly as they're supposed to. As a result, cells pile up, forming dry, red, scaly patches, especially on the elbows, scalp, knees, or torso.

Doctors still don't know what causes psoriasis. There is certainly a hereditary link, and the immune system may be involved as well. It isn't contagious and it isn't dangerous, but it can be unsightly. It also tends to get worse during times of stress or when the skin gets dry and irritated.

There isn't a cure for psoriasis, although it can often be controlled with medications. In addition, there at things you can do at home to keep the flare-ups from taking over.

WHEN TO SEE THE DOCTOR

Many people with psoriasis will only have small "problem areas" on their skin. But sometimes the scales are much more widespread, making the skin feel dry and itchy. When psoriasis is spreading and you're getting increasingly self-conscious, it's time to see a doctor. There are a number of prescription drugs, including steroids and methotrexate (a drug commonly used for arthritis), which can be very effective for getting this condition under control.

Soak up some sun. Nearly everyone with psoriasis tries to spend at least a few minutes a day in the sun. Research has shown that sunlight is very effective for reducing skin inflammation and scaling. If you live in a chilly northern clime and aren't able to bask in the sun's rays, your doctor may recommend that you treat your skin with artificial rays from a special lamp or a tanning booth.

Keep your skin moist. Using moisturizer on a regular basis is essential when you have psoriasis. You don't have to use anything fancy. Many people find that dabbing on a little petroleum jelly can help prevent skin cells from building up. Moisturizers that contain lactic acid can also be very effective. Moisturizers work best when they're applied right after bathing or showering, doctors say, because they help lock in moisture.

Make a soothing bath. Taking a long bath can soothe the itch of psoriasis temporarily, but it also dries out the skin. Doctors often advise adding a little colloidal oatmeal to the water, which will help your skin stay softer.

Mix some relief. During psoriasis flare-ups the skin can get extraordinarily itchy. For quick relief, mix about a quarter-cup of baking soda in a few quarts of water. Soak a towel in the mixture, wring it out, and apply it to your skin for a soothing compress. Adding vinegar instead of baking soda to the water will also calm the itch.

Don't drink alcohol. Doctors aren't sure why, but drinking alcohol often makes psoriasis worse. For some people, in fact, even a drink or two can put the skin into an uproar. You may want to try drinking less or even stop entirely for a few weeks to see if your symptoms improve.

RASHES

A rash is one of the most telltale signs that something is bothering your skin. When you're under stress, sick, or have had a close encounter with insects or poisonous plants, the skin may display its unhappiness for all the world to see, in the form of a red, itchy, irritating rash.

What can make some rashes so annoying is their sheer unpredictability. They can come out of the blue, leaving you (and your doctor) wondering what the heck caused them. But it often doesn't matter all that much. Most rashes are easy to treat regardless of the cause. Here are a few ways to keep your skin happy.

WHEN TO SEE THE DOCTOR

It's not common, but some rashes are a sign of serious medical problems, including sexually transmitted diseases, bacterial infections, or dangerous allergic reactions. You should call your doctor immediately if a rash doesn't go away within a day or two, or if it's deep-colored, oozing, or accompanied by other symptoms such as difficulty breathing, dizziness, or painful urination. You should also call your doctor if you've recently started taking a new medication and are getting a rash.

Bathe in cool water. Spending ten or fifteen minutes in a cool bath will often make rashes feel better and may help speed them on their way. Cool compresses are also effective. Don't bathe in hot water, however, because that will often make rashes worse.

Take comfort in tea. A traditional remedy for rashes is to brew a pot of chamomile or comfrey tea and use it to make a tea compress. Let it cool until it's comfortably warm. Then soak a towel or gauze pad in the tea and apply it to the rash for ten to fifteen minutes. You can repeat this treatment as often as necessary.

Turn down the heat. Rashes often occur during hot, humid weather. As its name implies, this is especially true of heat rash, which results in tiny pink bumps on the neck, upper back, or other parts of the body that get hot and sweaty. In most cases, this type of rash will disappear as soon as you've showered, dried off, and exposed the rash to air. It also helps to stay in air-conditioned areas or to use a fan, and to wear comfortable clothes that help keep moisture away from the skin.

Stop the inflammation. A very effective treatment for most rashes is to apply over-the-counter hydrocortisone cream. It helps stop inflammation and itching very quickly, and is very safe to use. Just be sure to ask your doctor or pharmacist if hydrocortisone is all right for the type of rash that you have.

Learn to relax. The skin is very sensitive to emotional changes. Doctors have found that people who experience the most stress are often the ones most likely to get rashes. To keep your skin calm, you have to keep your mind and emotions calm, as well. Doctors often recommend that people who get rashes take up meditation, yoga, or other activities that can reduce stress and help you feel calm and in control.

RECTAL ITCHING

Few sensations are more unpleasant than having an itch you can't reach. Rectal itching is even worse. You don't want to scratch in public. And even in private, scratching doesn't always help and often makes the itching worse.

Many things cause rectal itching, including hemorrhoids or irritation in the delicate tissues around the anus. Most of the time, however, it's easy to prevent or even stop entirely. Here are a few ways to get to the bottom of it.

Sit in a warm tub. One of the easiest ways to soothe rectal itching is simply to sit in a warm bath for awhile. Soaking cleanses the area and the warm water increases circulation, which will help you feel better. Since tissues around the anus may be raw or irritated, it's best to soak in plain water. Adding bath beads or oils to the water may make the irritation worse.

Douse it with witch hazel. This traditional remedy can be very soothing for an anal itch. Soak a cotton ball in witch hazel and apply it for a few seconds. You'll instantly feel a rush of cool relief. It's safe to apply witch hazel every few hours, or as often as necessary to ease the itch.

Put on some petroleum jelly. An itch where you sit may occur simply because the area is dry. Applying a little petroleum jelly will help moisturize the delicate anal lining and protect it from further irritation.

RESTLESS LEG SYNDROME

Moving your legs is great exercise, but most people do it during the day. For those with restless leg syndrome, however, the legs really get moving at night, and that can be a real problem.

Doctors aren't sure what causes restless leg syndrome, but the symptoms are well-known. Shortly after going to bed, people with this condition will begin having aches in their legs. Some people describe a pins-and-needles sensation. Others say they feel as though bugs are running around underneath the skin. The sensations can be maddening, and the only way to get relief is to twitch or kick the legs, or get up and walk around. And this can go on all night.

Restless leg syndrome isn't dangerous, but it can badly disrupt your sleep—as well as that of your bedmate. To keep your legs a little calmer, here's what doctors advise.

WHEN TO SEE THE DOCTOR

Even though restless leg syndrome usually isn't serious, the same symptoms may be caused by other conditions, such as Parkinson's disease. It's worth getting a checkup just to be sure nothing more serious is going on.

Move your legs during the day. Probably the best strategy for easing restless legs at night is to move your legs during the day. Doctors have found that people who walk, jog, or cycle daily often have fewer problems with restless legs than those who are more sedentary. Don't exercise immediately before bedtime, though, because that can make it harder to get to sleep.

Give your muscles a rub. When your legs are tingling at night, reach down and give them a vigorous massage. It won't prevent the problem, but it may ease the discomfort.

Teach your legs to relax. Some people have found that a technique called progressive relaxation, in which each of the body's muscles are relaxed one at a time, can help ease restless legs. Here's how it works. While you're lying in bed, breathe deeply for a few minutes. Then, starting at your feet and working upward to your head, tense each muscle for a few seconds, then relax slowly. Take your time. By the time you've reached the top of your head, your whole body will feel warm and relaxed—and your legs may be less restless, as well.

Take a warm bath. Taking a warm bath before bedtime can help ease the discomfort of restless legs. In fact, anything you can do to relax your body and mind may help your legs stay a little bit calmer.

Slow down on the stimulants. Drinking coffee or alcohol near bedtime can rev up your entire body, including the muscles and nerves in the legs. Doctors have found that some people with restless legs get significant relief when they give up coffee, cola, and other caffeine-containing foods and drinks.

SINUSITIS

A stuffy nose is bad enough, but what happens when the congestion is actually inside your head? This is what is behind a condition called sinusitis. The sinuses consist of mucus-lined hollow spaces—above and below the eyes and on each side of the nose. The sinuses normally drain quite easily. But when you have a cold or congestion due to allergies, the openings to the sinuses may get blocked, allowing mucus to accumulate. Eventually the sinuses may get infected, causing fever, headaches, and an unpleasant-tasting mucus that drips down the back of your throat. Doctors call this condition sinusitis.

Sinusitis has been called the number-one health complaint in America, affecting millions of people each year. In some cases, people with sinusitis need antibiotics to clear up the infection. More often, the condition will go away on its own within a week or two. Until it does, however, you may feel as though your entire head is under water. To loosen congestion and ease the pain, here are a few things you may want to try.

WHEN TO SEE THE DOCTOR

Sinusitis usually isn't serious. But if the congestion doesn't go away, or if the mucus is turning yellow or green, you may have a serious infection and you should call your doctor. Most of the time, antibiotics will clear up sinusitis in a hurry. In rare cases, a doctor may recommend surgery to clean out the sinuses so they'll drain more easily in the future.

Breathe some steam. The trick to relieving sinusitis is to unblock the openings so the mucus drains more freely.

The easiest way to do this is simply to breathe hot, humid air. Taking a hot shower, soaking in the tub or plugging in a room humidifier will help make the mucus watery so it drains more easily. For a more concentrated steam "bath" doctors sometimes recommend putting a pot of water on to boil. Remove it from the heat and lean over it, draping a towel around your head to trap the steam, and breathe deeply for a few minutes. Just don't get too close to the water or you could wind up scalded.

Soothe it with soup. Doctors often suggest that people with sinusitis put hot, spicy soup on the menu—not just for dinner, but all day long. Spicy foods act as natural decongestants, helping mucus drain. In addition, drinking hot liquids will loosen mucus in the throat and airways.

Even if you're not in the mood for soup, spicy foods can be very helpful. They contain a number of chemicals, including capsaicin, which stimulate nerves that trigger a runny nose. The more mucus is able to drain, the less stuffy your head will feel.

Raise your head. Some doctors recommend putting wood blocks under the head of your bed or propping yourself up with pillows at night. The natural process of gravity helps mucus drain.

Sniff some saline. Saline sprays, available at pharmacies, are very helpful at clearing mucus from the nose, which makes it easier for the sinuses to drain. You can make your own saline solution by putting a little bit of table salt in a cup of warm water and sniffing it out of your palm.

Tap a healthy solution. Drinking water is enormously helpful when you have sinusitis. Putting extra fluids in your body makes the mucus watery and more likely to drain. When you have sinusitis, doctors usually say to drink eight to twelve glasses of water a day, which, by the

139

way, is helpful for all kinds of conditions and your overall health maintenance.

Put away the cigarettes. People who smoke often have more trouble with sinusitis because smoking dries the nasal passages, making it harder for mucus and bacteria in the sinuses to drain out. By quitting smoking you will not only relieve the discomfort of sinusitis, but you will decrease your likelihood of getting it in the future.

Use a decongestant. When your head is throbbing, you may want to take a shortcut to relief by using an over-the-counter decongestant for a few days. These products shrink tissues, so they will produce less mucus.

SMOKING

It's hard to exaggerate the dangers of smoking. Cigarette smoke contains more than 4,000 chemicals, including such things as cyanide, arsenic, and formaldehyde. Doctors estimate that 400,000 Americans die every year from smoking-related illnesses. That's more than the number of deaths from alcohol, illegal drugs, and motor vehicle accidents combined. In the long run, cigarettes contribute to a vast number of health threats, including cancer, heart disease, and emphysema; as well as "minor" problems such as wrinkles.

Most people who smoke would like to quit. But as every smoker knows, quitting can be incredibly difficult. But here are a few tricks doctors advise.

WHEN TO SEE THE DOCTOR

Studies have shown that giving up cigarettes is one of the most difficult things to do. In fact, some experts believe it's harder to quit smoking than to give up addicting drugs. If you've repeatedly tried to quit without success, see your doctor. There are a number of medications—prescription as well as over-the-counter—that can help get the cravings under control. These are often in gum or patch form, making them easy to administer. In addition, your doctor may help you find a stop-smoking program. For many people, these programs are far more effective than trying to quit on their own.

Pick a quit date. It takes tremendous willpower to give up a habit that may have lasted for years or even decades. You have to make a solid commitment. One way to do this is to pick an exact date when you'll quit—a week from Tuesday, or on the first of the month. Before that date, tell everyone—your friends, colleagues, and family—when you plan to quit. Then go through with it. The more people you involve in your struggle, the more motivated you'll be to go through with it.

Avoid the triggers. Every smoker has certain activities— sipping a beer, sitting out on the deck, or chatting on the phone—that just don't seem the same without a cigarette. To break the habit, experts recommend avoiding the activities that you associate with smoking. Don't drink for a few weeks. Relax indoors instead of outside. Anything you can do to avoid "smoking behavior" will make it easier to give up the cigarettes for good.

Give yourself healthy alternatives. Just as some types of behavior increase the craving to smoke, others reduce it. Going for a jog, working in the garden, or even washing a sink-full of dishes will keep your hands and mind busy, so you're less likely to crave a cigarette.

Take five. Studies have shown that a cigarette craving

141

usually is most intense for about five minutes. If you can get through those five minutes—by taking a walk, for example, or keeping your hands busy doing something else—you'll find that the craving in the next five minutes and the five minutes after that will be much less intense.

Nip it in the bud. Cats don't smoke, but they certainly know the value of a little catnip. Alternative practitioners have found that drinking catnip tea can reduce feelings of nervousness and tension, making it easier to give up smoking. Other herbal teas that have a calming effect include skullcap and valerian.

Drink a little milk. For some reason, drinking milk gives cigarette smoke an unpleasant taste. Many people who have successfully quit made it a point to drink milk throughout the day, which helped reduce the cravings.

Make smoking difficult. If you've been trying to quit, but haven't quite succeeded, you can improve your chances in the future by limiting the places where you allow yourself to smoke. For starters, you may want to quit smoking in the car. Even if you only drive a few miles a day, this will allow you to cut back by a few cigarettes a day. Don't let yourself smoke in the house, either. When it's twenty degrees outside and the wind is blowing, you may find that you really don't want to have another cigarette just yet. It's not as good as quitting, but it will lower your dependence and make it easier to quit entirely another day.

SNEEZING

It's not painful or socially unacceptable. It's not even annoying—if you do it occasionally. But when your "achoos" are coming on cue, you know there's too much sneezing going on.

Sneezing is your body's way of cleaning out the nasal passages and discharging irritating particles like dust or pollen. But when you have a cold or allergies, non-stop sneezing can make your nasal passages sore and irritated. Some people even get nosebleeds from non-stop sneezing. To give your nose a break, here's what doctors recommend.

Neutralize the problem with nettle. This herbal remedy has been shown to ease inflammation in the nasal passages and help reduce congestion that can lead to sneezing. Some people make nettle teas, but an easier solution is to take nettle supplements, available at health food stores. Following the directions on the label, you can take them whenever your nose starts getting a little twitchy.

Pour a glass of orange juice. Along with citrus fruits and a variety of fruits and vegetables, orange juice is very rich in vitamin C, which may help relieve sneezing by reducing the amount of histamine your body releases.

Put more vegetables on the menu. Along with fruits, many vegetables are rich sources of bioflavonoids. These are natural chemicals, which, like vitamin C, can curtail the body's production of sneeze-causing histamine.

Sneeze-proof your home. Your best natural remedy against sneezing is to scrub your house clean of allergens. Doctors recommend vacuuming, mopping, and dusting as

143

often as possible, which will help eliminate the dust that causes sneezing. It's also a good idea to scour bathrooms and basements, which often harbor large amounts of sneeze-causing molds. You may even want to wash rugs, pillows, and even stuffed animals once a week to wash away allergy-causing particles before they cause problems.

Clean your mattresses and bedding. Evidence has shown that microscopic skin flakes, called dander, often cause sneezing and other allergy symptoms. The best way to get rid of these particles is to wash your sheets and pillow cases once a week. Many people find that covering the mattress with a plastic cover and wiping it down once a week will also help stop sneezing.

Give your cat a bath. Millions of people are allergic to cats—and, less often, to dogs. Studies have shown that washing your pet once a week can dramatically decrease the amount of sneeze-causing allergens that get into the air—and, of course, into your nose. At the very least you may want to keep your pets out of the bedroom. Spending even just eight hours a day away from their allergy-causing particles may help you sneeze less often the rest of the time.

Take antihistamines. These over-the-counter medicines are very effective at blocking your body's production of histamine. You don't want to take them all the time, but if your sneezing is seasonal—as it often is in people with allergies—taking antihistamines during flare-ups will give you some much-needed relief.

SNORING

Everyone snores occasionally, and some people do it a lot. But when your spouse is thinking about moving into the next room and the neighbors are pounding the walls, it may be time to turn down the noise.

Snoring occurs when loose tissues in the upper airways, which normally sag a bit when you lie down, start rattling around when you breathe. The problem is worse when you're overweight, because there is more tissue in the throat that can partially block the flow of air. Drinking alcohol also increases snoring—both the frequency and volume—as do many sleep problems.

You can't stop snoring entirely, but there are ways to reduce the frequency and also make it less noisy. Here's how.

WHEN TO SEE THE DOCTOR

Snoring that is unusually loud or is accompanied by wheezing or gasping sounds may be a sign of sleep apnea, a potentially serious sleep problem in which people literally stop breathing during the night. Sleep apnea is most common among older, overweight men, although women can get it, too. If you or your spouse is periodically gasping for breath during the night, it's important to call your doctor. Without treatment, sleep apnea can lead to fatigue, headaches, or even high blood pressure and heart problems.

Slim down. This is perhaps the most effective way to turn down the volume on snoring. When you're overweight, it's a lot harder for air to squeeze through fatty tissue in the throat and airways, which can lead to wall-shaking snores. Doctors have found that losing even a few pounds can be very effective for reducing snoring.

145

Prop yourself up. When you lie flat on your back, tissues in the throat naturally fall into the air passages. Many people find they can reduce snoring simply by propping themselves up at night with a pillow or two. Better yet, sleep on your side, which makes it easier to breathe than when you're lying on your back.

Try the tennis ball trick. The problem with sleeping on your side is that during the night you may flip over on your back and start snoring again. Some doctors recommend sewing a little pouch on the back of your pajama top or a T-shirt and putting a tennis ball inside. Then, if you roll over on your back during sleep, the ball will make you uncomfortable, so you'll naturally roll back into a snore-free position—usually without being aware of it.

Avoid that nightcap. Drinking alcohol is a very common cause of snoring because it makes tissues in the airways more flaccid. You don't have to give up alcohol entirely, but you should avoid it after dinner or late in the evening, when it is most likely to have an effect on your sleep and snoring.

Ask about medications. If you're taking sleeping pills, antihistamines, or other medications, ask your doctor if they might be contributing to the problem. Any medication that makes you sleep can potentially increase your snoring, as well.

Don't get overtired. Doctors have found that not getting enough sleep in general can increase snoring when you finally do hit the hay. Keeping a regular sleep schedule will help you sleep a little more soundly and with a lot less noise.

Exercise often. Evidence suggests that staying in shape and getting regular exercise can help improve muscle tone inside the airways as well as elsewhere in the body. And exercising makes you less likely to become congested, which will also help reduce snoring.

SORE THROAT

Your throat is only about six to eight inches long, but when it's raw and burning it can feel like it goes on for mile after painful mile.

A sore throat usually means you have a cold or the flu. It can also be caused by dry air, pollution, or simply hooting and hollering too loud at a football game. When you're sick, of course, it may take a few days before your throat is entirely back to normal. But there are many ways to get quick relief.

WHEN TO SEE THE DOCTOR

It's important to call your doctor when your throat stays sore—or is getting worse—for more than a few days. You should also call your doctor if your sore throat is accompanied by other symptoms such as fever, achy joints, or a rash, or if you've lost your voice.

Reach for tea and honey. Every grandmother knows this remedy. Any warm beverage can make a sore throat feel better, but tea is especially good because it contains compounds called tannins, which can ease the irritation. Adding honey to tea will coat your throat with a soft, soothing, protective layer. Try caffeine-free herbal teas for soothing relief.

147

Get more vitamin C. The body uses vitamin C for wound healing, and getting more of this nutrient when you have a sore, scratchy throat may help it to heal more quickly. The Recommended Daily Value for vitamin C is sixty milligrams. But when you have a sore throat because of a cold or the flu, many doctors recommend getting more—up to 500 or 1,000 milligrams a day.

Have a soothing gargle. This traditional remedy can be very effective. Add a teaspoon of salt to a cup of warm water and gargle away. You'll get relief almost instantly, and you can repeat this as often as it seems to help.

Breathe soothing moisture. A sore throat is usually a dry, scratchy throat. Breathing in moisture—either by taking a long steamy shower or simply plugging in a humidifier—will help protect the delicate linings inside the throat and make them less irritated.

Pause for a moment of silence. Giving your voice a rest will help ease a sore throat by reducing strain on the vocal cords. You don't have to take a vow of silence, but simply talking less—and not shouting—for a few days can make a big difference.

Take some aspirin. One reason throats get sore is that the irritated tissues get inflamed and swollen. Taking aspirin will help reduce the inflammation, and also help block the production of chemicals in the body that contribute to the pain. Don't give aspirin to children with sore throats, however, because it increases the risk for a serious neurological problem called Reye's Syndrome. Children should be given acetaminophen, such as Tylenol, instead.

SPLINTERS

The amazing thing about splinters is that something so small can hurt so much. You can't ignore them because they often get infected and hurt even more. And getting them out by digging with a needle often makes things worse. To remove splinters without the pain, here's what doctors advise.

Soak your skin. Before removing a splinter, it's a good idea to soak the area in warm water for ten or fifteen minutes. Water makes the wood softer and also causes it to swell. In some cases this will cause the splinter to pop out on its own. Even when it doesn't, it's much easier to remove a splinter when the skin is soft and pliable.

Grease it out. One traditional technique for removing splinters is to smear on a little bit of bacon fat and then cover it with an adhesive strip. In a day or two, the splinter will often be gone. Bacon fat contains a lot of salt, which draws moisture from the skin, and may draw the splinter out, as well.

Apply a little ice. To quickly ease the pain of a splinter, apply an ice cube for a few minutes. This will help numb the area, making the splinter easier to remove.

Spray on some relief. Another way to numb the pain is to give the area a spritz with an over-the-counter first aid spray. As a bonus, these sprays will help disinfect the area so it's less likely to get infected.

149

Use the right tweezers. It's not always easy to get a grip on a splinter with tweezers. You'll have better success if you use tweezers that have ridges or grooves on the end, which will improve their grip strength. Begin by sterilizing the tweezers with a little rubbing alcohol. Grab the splinter as close to the skin as possible and pull firmly. Do your best to remove the splinter at the same angle as it entered the skin, which will help prevent it from breaking off inside. When you're done, swab a little rubbing alcohol on the skin to disinfect it, or at least wash the area well with soap and water.

SPRAINS

When you slip on the ice or step off a curb the wrong way, you can put tremendous strain on one or more of your body's ligaments—those tough cords that bind bones together. This causes the ligaments to stretch as far as they comfortably can—and then a little more. It's that "little more" that doctors refer to as muscle sprains.

Sprains can be incredibly painful, and they're often slow to heal. There may be swelling around the area, and in some cases there will be a bruise, as well. When you've sprained a muscle you may want to see your doctor just to make sure you haven't seriously injured a joint. Most of the time, however, sprains are easy to treat at home—as long as you're not in too much of a hurry to be up and about again.

Put it on ice. The most important thing you can do for a sprain is to ice it as soon as possible. Applying cold for fifteen to twenty minutes soon after the injury will help prevent swelling and pain, and also will help it get better more quickly.

Give it some pressure and raise it high. After using ice, it's a good idea to put pressure on a muscle sprain—by wrapping it with an Ace bandage, for example—to reduce swelling. In addition, you should elevate the area higher than your heart, which will reduce the amount of blood flowing to the area.

Apply some heat. Although applying cold for the first twenty-four hours is the best way to prevent swelling, many people find that applying heat the next day is also very soothing. Taking a hot bath is the easiest way to ease a sprain. Or you can apply a hot water bottle or a heating pad to the area. Applying heat increases circulation, which can help speed healing.

Get some new shoes. Of all sprains, 85 percent occur when the ankle turns inward. It's important to wear shoes that provide good ankle support. If you're an athlete, replacing your shoes frequently will give your ankles all the support they need.

STOMACHACHES

Perhaps you had a few too many helpings at that Thanksgiving buffet. Or maybe you haven't eaten all day and your stomach is letting you know it isn't happy. Regardless of the cause—eating too much, not enough, or even being too stressed—a stomachache can make you feel as though there's a vise closing on your midsection.

The best "remedy" for most stomachaches is to simply wait until they get better on their own. When you need quicker relief, here are some helpful tips.

WHEN TO SEE THE DOCTOR

When you have a stomachache as well as other symptoms, like vomiting, diarrhea, fever, or a rash, see your doctor right away. There could be a more serious underlying problem, like appendicitis, that's causing the pain, and you need to get it checked out right away.

Reach for a light snack. When your stomach is hurting and you haven't been eating, having a snack is often the quickest way to ease the pain. Food in your stomach will absorb excess stomach acid, which often causes aches. Good snacks include toasted wheat bread with a little honey or some unsalted crackers. Bland snacks are best. This isn't the time to be eating four-alarm chili or acidic foods like citrus fruits or tomatoes.

Have a piece of fruit. With the exception of citrus, fresh fruits are often very soothing for a stomachache. They help absorb stomach acid while also putting more dietary fiber in your system. Experts have found that fiber-rich snacks are more effective at stopping stomachaches than those that don't contain fiber.

Try an herbal remedy. Herbal teas made from chamomile, catnip, or fennel have been used for centuries for easing digestive complaints, and many doctors believe they really are very helpful.

Take an antacid. Over-the-counter antacids neutralize stomach acids that may cause stomach pain. It doesn't really matter which kind you buy. Antacids that are high in magnesium are often recommended if you also have diarrhea because they're slightly constipating. Those containing sodium bicarbonate won't cause constipation, but may cause gas in some people.

Use bubbles for stomach troubles. Stomachaches may be caused by trapped gas in the stomach. To get it out, some doctors recommend having a glass of cola or another soda—or that old standby, Alka-Seltzer. Carbonated drinks will often make you burp—and when you do, the gas is out.

Move around a little. Studies have shown that exercise can help make your digestive system work more efficiently, which is often all it takes to help ease stomach pain. In addition, exercise is an excellent strategy for relieving stress, which is a common cause of midsection misery.

STRESS

Most of us are experts at stress—at getting it, not getting rid of it. Stress spares no one, and many doctors believe it's the greatest health threat facing Americans today. We read about stress in newspapers and magazines and watch programs about it on television. But the more we learn about stress, the more stressed we get.

Stress is a natural part of life, of course, and you can't get rid of it entirely. Nor would you want to, because some stress is good. The excitement of seeing old friends, going to a party, or starting a new job you've been looking forward to—these are good kinds of stress that can keep you motivated and excited. But a lot of stress isn't so positive. When you're worried about life, stress can make you tired and depressed. It saps your strength and keeps you awake at nights. It can even make you sick. Some studies suggest that at least two-thirds of visits to doctors are related to stress.

It's impossible to avoid stressful situations or emotions. What you can do, however, is learn to put stress in perspective so that it doesn't take over your life. Here's what doctors advise.

WHEN TO SEE THE DOCTOR

Everyone has different "comfort levels" when it comes to coping with stress. It's up to you to recognize when the stress in your life is too much to handle alone. If you're experiencing stress every day, or if you're getting sick much more often than you used to, it's time to call your doctor or a professional counselor. In many cases, getting therapy or even taking medications will make it much easier for you to control stress rather than having it control you.

Identify the problems. One of the reasons stress often seems so unmanageable is that it's hard to put your finger on what, exactly, is bothering you. Suppose, for example, your stress level starts rising on Sunday nights. You know you're bothered about your job, but what part of your job? Are you in your boss's bad graces? Is a project giving you trouble? Do you have to give a speech in a few weeks? Until you identify the real source of your stress, you can't begin to cope with it.

Doctors often recommend making a list of everything that gives you stress, from the most mundane and minor to the most serious. Use as much paper as you need. When you're done, you may be surprised to learn just how much stress there really is in your life. More importantly, you'll now know some of the things you need to watch out for, and this will help you feel more in control.

Keep things in perspective. When you have made a list of all the different stresses in your life, try to put them in perspective. Which are truly serious and which are mainly annoying? Of those that are serious, ask yourself just how serious they really are. Some things that seem serious at first may not seem so bad when you put them in perspective. Some people make a point of asking themselves, "Will this really matter a year from now?" When the answer is "no," you'll know that what you're dealing with is really a short-term problem, and that no matter how bad things seem now, you're going to get through it—probably a lot quicker than you think.

Get lots of exercise. Doctors agree that physical exercise is one of your strongest allies in the fight against stress. Exercise literally trains your body to cope with all sorts of stress—by strengthening the heart and lungs and by stimulating the release of chemicals in the brain that make you

155

feel calmer and more in control. Exercise also boosts confidence, which is invaluable when you're fighting stress.

You don't have to be a hard-core athlete to "train" against stress. In fact, you don't have to be an athlete at all. Doctors agree that even mild exercise—walking several times a week, for example—will help strengthen all your defenses, including those that are essential for stopping stress.

Put your mind to work. Evidence suggests that you can fight stress simply by harnessing the power of your mind. With a technique called visualization, in which you imagine yourself triumphing over stress, you can actually change the chemistry in your brain, giving yourself more confidence and making it easier to fight whatever life throws at you.

The trick to visualization is to perceive your stress in a visual way. Suppose, for example, you imagine stress as being an elevator at the top of a building. In your mind, imagine that the elevator is gradually, slowly coming down, and, as it does, your levels of stress are coming down as well. Take your time. The more thoroughly you create this image in your mind, the more real it will seem. By the time the elevator finally reaches the ground, you'll know that your stress has come down with it. You may find that you feel calmer than you did before.

Get a massage. Massage has been around for thousands of years, and even the ancient Egyptians, Greeks, and Romans knew of its restorative powers. Massage improves blood circulation, reduces muscle tension, stimulates the nervous system, reduces pain and swelling, and aids digestion. It can be incredibly powerful for rejuvenating your mind and spirit and reducing stress.

Take a "mental minute." One of the reasons stress is so rampant is that many of us hardly ever find time to relax.

Yet relaxation has been shown to be incredibly powerful for stopping stress. And you don't have to spend your entire weekend at the beach (although that would be nice) to get the benefits. Many doctors recommend a strategy called "meditative breathing," in which you concentrate on your breathing for as little as twenty or thirty seconds. Several times a day, breathe in deeply and hold it for a second. Then slowly breathe out, focusing all your mental energy on your breathing. It sounds easy, and it is. Doing this regularly will create a breathing space between your emotions and your troubles. At the same time, this sort of concentrated breathing floods your body with oxygen, which will strengthen your entire body and make it better able to handle stress.

De-stress with nutrition. One of the most intriguing findings of stress research is that what you eat can play a direct role in causing—or reducing—stress. People who are low in the B vitamins, for example, will often feel more anxious or depressed than folks who get enough. The same is true of vitamin C and other nutrients. You don't have to load up on supplements to get the benefits of vitamins, although your doctor may recommend that you take one or more of them. For most people, simply eating plenty of fruits, vegetables, whole grains, and legumes will provide an abundance of these "mood-boosting" vitamins.

Count on carbohydrates. Doctors aren't sure why, but many people are able to help control stress by eating less fat and more carbohydrates, which are found in foods like pasta, cereals, and bread. Carbohydrates produce quick, long-lasting energy that can help you feel more in control. In addition, your body uses carbohydrates to create the brain chemicals that have been shown to lower stress.

157

SUNBURN

Getting sunburned is a lot like doing your taxes. No one ever thinks about it until it's too late—and by then your skin is nearly the color of a ripe tomato, and it feels like it's on fire.

Sunburns are more than just painful. Research has shown that getting even one sunburn in your life can significantly increase your risk for cancer. In addition, long-term sun exposure causes the skin to lose its elasticity, making it look rougher and more wrinkled later on.

It can be hard to resist the lure of the sun. Even when you're trying to be cautious you may occasionally get a few more rays than you intended. To put out the fire fast, here's what doctors advise.

WHEN TO SEE THE DOCTOR

When you've fallen asleep on the beach and your skin feels hot enough to fry an egg, you may have more than a simple sunburn. Like any burn, some sunburns can be extremely serious, damaging multiple layers of skin and even burning tissues underneath. If you have a sunburn and are also having chills, nausea, dizziness, or fever, you should see a doctor right away. You should also see a doctor if your burn blisters or swells. It's not common, but serious sunburns may cause internal problems that need immediate medical care.

Give your skin a drink. One of the most effective healing secrets for sunburn is also one of the simplest: Take a cool shower or bath. Flooding your hot, burning skin with cool water will quickly turn down the temperature, stopping the burn before it does more damage.

Add some vinegar. Another way to soothe a sunburn is to add a cup of white vinegar to bath water. Vinegar baths are very soothing and will help relieve pain in a hurry. If you don't have any vinegar, add a cup of baking soda to the water, or even a dozen or so drops of "essential oils," like chamomile or lavender.

Use a moisturizer. Spending time in the sun quickly robs the skin of its protective moisture, which is why sunburns are so painful. After bathing or showering, do your skin a favor and rub in a generous amount of moisturizer. This will help replace the moisture that the sun's burning rays took out.

Put aloe to work. Another way to moisturize the skin and ease sunburn is to rub on a coating of gel from an aloe vera leaf. Studies have shown that aloe vera is very effective for helping burns heal more quickly. You can buy aloe vera lotions, but many doctors believe that the natural gel from the plant works best. You can also buy pure gel from your local pharmacy.

Try a milk compress. Many people with sunburn have gotten quick relief by soaking a towel in milk and applying it to the burn for about half an hour. Milk contains a lot of natural fats, which will help soothe the burn. Just be sure to rinse your skin thoroughly when you're done to remove the milk.

Stop the pain and swelling. Taking aspirin or ibuprofen will help stop the pain of sunburn from the inside out. These medications not only ease pain, but will also help reduce inflammation, which lets skin heal more quickly.

Put on protection. The fortunate thing about sunburn is that it's almost always easy to prevent. When you're going to be spending time outdoors, take a minute to rub on a sunscreen with an SPF (sun-protection factor) of fifteen or higher. You can even buy facial moisturizers that include sunscreen as one of the ingredients.

159

SWIMMER'S EAR

Children get it frequently. So do dogs that splash in ponds and lakes. Even taking a dip in the neighborhood pool can set the stage for a painful and occasionally serious infection called swimmer's ear.

Swimmer's ear, or external otitis, occurs when bacteria or other organisms that live in water take up residence inside your ear. The warm, moist environment is entirely to their liking, and sometimes they'll thrive, causing a painful infection. Incidentally, you don't have to swim to get swimmer's ear. Anything that causes the insides of the ears to get moist—taking a shower, wearing a hearing aid, or even having too much ear wax can make it easy for the organisms to flourish.

It's usually not that difficult to stop swimmer's ear in its tracks. Here are a few things to try.

WHEN TO SEE THE DOCTOR

You can often treat swimmer's ear at home, but if the infection doesn't go away or starts getting worse you need to call your doctor. Some symptoms to watch for are a lot of pain and a discharge from the ear. Your doctor probably will give you a prescription for antibiotics, which knock out most ear infections within a week or two.

Start with a kitchen cure. Research has shown that garlic can kill a variety of germs, including those that cause swimmer's ear. When your ears start aching, squeeze a clove of garlic into a little bit of olive oil and apply a few drops to your ears. There's a good chance this will kill the germs before they have time to cause a full-blown infection.

Add some vinegar. Another way to help kill germs in the ear is with a few drops of white vinegar mixed half-and-half with rubbing alcohol. Put the drops in your ears, then tilt your head to let the fluid run out. This can be very helpful, but the rubbing alcohol may be painful if your ears are irritated. An alternative is to mix the vinegar with a few drops of water.

Dry your ears. Since the germs that cause swimmer's ear thrive in moisture, you can make your ears less hospitable simply by drying them out. After swimming, tilt your head to the side and pull on your ear to let the water out. Then put in a few drops of rubbing alcohol, which acts as a drying agent.

TEMPOROMANDIBULAR JOINT DISORDER (TMD)

Your jaw is hinged to the skull with two joints called the temporomandibular joints. As you would expect, these joints are nearly in perpetual motion. Every time you talk, chew gum, eat a sandwich, or even tense your jaw, these joints are hard at work. Over time this can lead to sore muscles, headaches, or even damaged cartilage or bone in the joints themselves. Doctors call this temporomandibular joint disorder, or TMD.

TMD can be excruciatingly painful, but in most cases it can be treated in the same way you would treat any other joint condition. Here's how.

WHEN TO SEE THE DOCTOR

Some people with TMD experience so much pain that they can barely open their mouths. Untreated, severe TMD can literally destroy the jaw joints. So it is critical to call your doctor if you're having jaw pain that's severe or seems to be getting worse. You also should get help if you're hearing loud popping or grinding sounds when you move your jaw.

Start with aspirin. Along with ibuprofen, aspirin is one of the best things you can take for the pain of TMD. It quickly reduces the swelling and also helps to block the production of chemicals in the body that are responsible for causing pain.

Give your jaw a break. When your jaw is aching you need to give it a rest. Talk as little as possible and try to avoid foods that require a lot of chewing. You should also retire the gum, since chewing gum can put enormous strain on the joints in the jaw.

Hang up on bad phone habits. You wouldn't think that how you hold the phone could affect your jaw, but it does. Doctors have found that people who cradle the telephone between their shoulders and ears while their hands are busy may have problems with TMD.

Rest your shoulders. Here's another unexpected cause of TMD: carrying a heavy handbag. Women who tend to carry purses or briefcases with the strap over a shoulder may be throwing their posture out of alignment, which can lead to jaw problems later on. If you can, switch to a lighter handbag, or at least alternate shoulders when you're carrying your purse around.

162

Cool it down. For temporary flare-ups of TMD, applying a cold pack or some ice cubes wrapped in a towel can be very soothing. If ice isn't nice, you may want to try applying a hot water bottle or a warm-towel compress, instead.

Watch those stressful habits. When stress levels rise our mouths go to work—chewing pens, fingernails, or gum. But when you have TMD, all that jaw action will only make the problem worse. There isn't an easy solution for stress, of course, but you may want to find some other way of working off the tension—one that doesn't involve moving your jaw. The best tension reducer? Exercise. The more you move your body, the less stress you'll feel.

TINNITUS

When you're hearing bells and it's not even Sunday, you could have tinnitus, an unusual symptom that causes a ringing, buzzing, or hissing sound in the ears. This is an especially persistent condition and it shouldn't be taken lightly.

WHEN TO SEE THE DOCTOR

People with tinnitus sometimes have an underlying problem, such an ear infection, Meniere's disease, or even heart disease or anemia. That's why people with tinnitus need to see a doctor as soon as possible.

In the meantime, however, there are ways to make tinnitus a little less annoying.

Stay away from stimulants. Doctors have found that drinking alcohol or coffee or smoking cigarettes can make tinnitus worse. For some people, giving these things up can significantly reduce the noise.

163

Stop taking aspirin. If you take aspirin regularly, you may want to consider switching to another pain reliever, like ibuprofen. Taking aspirin on a regular basis has been shown to increase the risk for tinnitus and also to make the symptoms worse.

Protect your ears. Exposure to loud sounds—everything from rock concerts to lawnmowers—can make tinnitis worse. Try to avoid loud environments whenever possible. Or, if like most people you can't do that, wearing ear plugs will significantly reduce the volume. You can purchase different types at a drugstore, or a doctor can prescribe something that will filter out harmful noise while still allowing you to hear.

Turn on a distraction. Having constant noise in your ears can be annoying, to say the least. Doctors often recommend that people "mask" the sound of tinnitus by giving themselves other things to listen to—playing the radio softly at night, for example, or even turning on a fan or a "white noise" machine.

Eat well to protect your hearing. Research suggests that a healthy diet may help protect you from tinnitus and other types of hearing damage. You may want to ask your doctor about magnesium, as well. Some research suggests that people who don't get enough of this mineral may be at risk for hearing problems.

URINARY INCONTINENCE

It's not a problem people like to discuss, even with their doctors. But urinary incontinence, in which the bladder occasionally loses control, is extremely common. Doctors estimate that about 10 percent of elderly people have this problem to some extent, and it's much more common in women than in men. There are many things that can cause it, including urinary tract infections, prostate problems, or even side effects from some medications.

Incontinence is usually easy to treat. The problem is that many people are too embarrassed to get help, and so they live with it, year after year. It doesn't have to be this way. In most cases, you can control or even stop incontinence entirely with simple home care. Here's what experts advise.

WHEN TO SEE THE DOCTOR

No matter how old you are, you shouldn't be losing bladder control. If you are, there's almost certainly something wrong and you should call your doctor. In addition to a general checkup, doctors usually take a urine sample to test for infections and other problems. They may also recommend x-rays or other tests to see if there's something going on inside that could be causing it. Your doctor may recommend medications that will help strengthen the "holding power" of the bladder.

Listen to nature's call. Many people go to the bathroom only when their bladder is sending out loud emergency signals—and then it may be too late. A better strategy is to set a "bathroom schedule" and stick with it—for example, going to the bathroom every hour even when you don't feel like you need to.

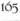

Of course, no one wants to go to the bathroom every hour on the hour. After a while, you won't have to. By "training" your bladder to expect regular relief, you can gradually increase the time between bathroom trips. Your goal is to be going every three or four hours eventually. As long as you stick to a regular schedule, your bladder will start making the adjustment.

Plan ahead. When you're going out, always visit the bathroom before you leave the house and again before you come back home. Urinating often will help to keep your bladder empty, so it's less likely to take you by surprise.

Strengthen your muscles. Urinary incontinence often occurs because the muscles that control the flow of urine aren't as strong as they could be. To get them back in shape, doctors recommend exercises known as Kegels. They're very easy to do. By regularly squeezing and relaxing the muscles that control the flow of urine—they're the same muscles you'd use to hold back a bowel movement—you'll make them stronger and less likely to "slip."

The good thing about Kegels is that you can do them anywhere and anytime—when you're doing the dishes, for example, or watching a movie. All you have to do is squeeze and relax those muscles ten times, rest for a moment, then do them ten more times. Repeating this three times every day will quickly get them back in shape.

Watch what you eat. Doctors have found that a number of foods, including tomatoes, spices, chocolate, and citrus fruits, can sometimes increase the risk of incontinence. Everyone responds to different foods differently, so you may want to keep track of what you're eating for a few weeks. That way you can see if there's a link between your diet and episodes of incontinence. If there is, you'll have a better idea of what you need to avoid in the future.

Give up cigarettes. Smoking can trigger incontinence in two ways. Nicotine has been shown to irritate the bladder, which may cause problems in some people. In addition, smoking often causes people to cough, and coughing jars the bladder, which is the last thing you need when you're trying to control incontinence.

VAGINAL DRYNESS

Along with gray hair, hot flashes, and irregular periods, vaginal dryness is a natural change that many women experience as they get older, due to declining levels of estrogen. But even though it's natural, it isn't any fun. It can make lovemaking difficult or even painful. And it's emotionally troubling to realize that what used to happen naturally is now something you have to think—and worry—about.

Doctors often recommend hormone replacement therapy for women in or approaching menopause. By increasing the amount of estrogen in the body, this will often help reverse vaginal dryness. But even if you don't take estrogen, there are ways to manage this condition at home. Here's how.

Take advantage of lubricants. There are many lubricants that can help relieve vaginal dryness. Doctors recommend using lubricants that are water-based, like K-Y Jelly or Astroglide. But you should avoid oil-based lubricants. They can be irritating and may upset the vagina's natural chemical balance.

167

Put fish on the menu. Along with sunflower seeds, fish contain fatty acids, which have been shown to help the body retain estrogen.

Give yourself more time. As women get older the body naturally takes longer to prepare for sex. One of the best "remedies" for vaginal dryness is simply to slow down and allow more time for foreplay.

WHEN TO SEE THE DOCTOR

Vaginal dryness isn't always a "harmless" change caused by menopause. If the dryness is accompanied by bleeding, itching, or pain, there may be underlying problems, such as an infection, which need to be taken care of. You should play it safe and see your doctor right away.

VARICOSE VEINS

They usually don't hurt. They don't cause disease. And about two-thirds of women and half of all men have them. They're so common, in fact, that many experts say they're no more of a medical problem than having freckles.

But varicose veins are a problem for some people, if only because they can mark the surface of the skin with lacy (and occasionally bumpy) networks of red or blue veins. Varicose veins occur when tiny valves in the veins that normally keep blood flowing toward the heart weaken or collapse. This can cause blood to pool inside the veins. When enough blood accumulates, the veins begin to swell or even break, causing varicose veins. Anyone can get them, but they often occur during pregnancy or as a result of being overweight, when increases in pressure damage the vein walls.

WHEN TO SEE THE DOCTOR

When varicose veins are extremely large—or when certain large veins deep inside the legs are affected—doctors sometimes recommend surgery to remove them. More often, the best care is home care.

Put your feet up. What better way is there to end your day than by putting your feet up? Raising your legs above the level of the heart will allow gravity to help pull blood out of the leg veins and send it toward the heart. This will often reduce swelling as well as aches, doctors say.

Give your legs a rest. People who spend all day standing, like waitresses or cashiers, often have trouble with varicose veins because standing makes it harder for blood to return to the heart. You'll do your legs a favor by getting off your feet and sitting down whenever you can.

Or keep them on the move. Even though standing still can make varicose veins worse, walking around or climbing stairs often makes them better because flexing muscles in your legs helps the veins work more efficiently at moving blood along.

Take one in the morning and one at night. Aspirin is often recommended as a "blood thinner" and it may help people with varicose veins. Ask your doctor if taking one aspirin every morning and another one at night will help the blood flow more freely and if it is safe for you.

Break the habit. Smoking cigarettes causes blood vessels to constrict, making it harder for the blood to get through. There's some evidence that giving up cigarettes may help reduce the risk of varicose veins.

169

Give your legs some support. They're not for everyone, but for some people, support stockings can be very helpful. Available from pharmacies and physicians, the stockings put pressure on the legs and veins, which helps prevent blood from pooling.

Check your weight. If you've been putting on weight lately, your legs may be paying the price. People who are overweight are more likely to get varicose veins simply because they have more pressure in their legs that can weaken the veins.

WARTS

Over the centuries toads have been blamed for everything from droughts to curses, but warts are one thing they shouldn't have to take the rap for.

Warts are caused by a virus, which builds a little "house"—the wart—to keep itself comfortable. What's nice and cozy for the virus, however, isn't so attractive on the skin. Warts usually aren't painful, although the ones that can form on the bottom of your feet or on your fingertips can cause irritating pressure.

Most warts will disappear on their own, although it may take months or even years before they're gone. To speed things along, here's what you can do.

Put on a little tape. Some people find that covering a wart with adhesive tape for a few weeks will cause it to disappear—presumably because the tape keeps the wart moist and cuts off its oxygen supply. It's important, however, to change the tape once a week and to air out the area periodically to keep your skin healthy.

Apply some vitamin A. Evidence suggests that applying liquid vitamin A to the wart every day for two weeks can cause it to disappear. Doctors recommend buying vitamin A capsules, pricking the end with a pin, and squeezing the liquid on the wart.

Imagine them vanishing. Researchers have found that some people can literally make their warts disappear by spending several minutes a day mentally visualizing that they're shrinking or even crying for mercy. It sounds kooky, but doing this once or twice a day may help warts disappear more quickly.

Apply a wart remedy. There are a number of safe, effective wart-removal products that you can get from pharmacies. Most of these products contain mild acids that wear away the wart over a period of weeks.

WRINKLES

You don't see it happening, but one day you look in the mirror and realize that your face is showing the passage of time. As we get older, the skin naturally loses some of its elasticity, so it doesn't "snap back" the way it used to. In addition, a lifetime of sunshine and the downward pull of gravity also play a role in causing wrinkles.

You can't turn back the clock, but there are ways to keep your skin smoother. Here are a few tips you'll want to try.

Revitalize your skin with moisturizer. The skin naturally gets a little drier with age, making it less elastic and prone to wrinkles. Applying a moisturizer every day will help keep the skin soft and flexible. In addition, it can actually plump up the skin a bit, making wrinkles you already have less noticeable. You can apply moisturizers any time, but they work best when used on damp skin after a bath or shower, when they lock in extra moisture.

Add moisture from the inside out. Drinking eight to twelve glasses of water every day will help keep your entire body, including the vulnerable tissues in your skin, moist and healthy.

Block the rays. This is by far the most effective way there is to prevent wrinkles. Sunshine breaks down collagen, the substance in your skin that makes it supple and elastic. It also causes your skin to become thicker and tougher. Doctors recommend avoiding the sun as much as possible. When you go outside, be sure to wear sunscreen with a sun-protection factor (SPF) of fifteen or higher, which will block the damaging rays.

Put on some shades. The area around the eyes is very prone to wrinkles. Wearing your sunglasses whenever you go outdoors will cause you to squint less, which help's prevent "crow's feet" from forming.

Stock up on vitamins. Research has shown that vitamins A, C, and E may play a powerful role in protecting the skin. These nutrients are known as antioxidants because they block the effects of harmful oxygen molecules that damage tissues throughout the body, including in the skin. Eating fruits, vegetables, whole grains, nuts, and legumes will provide large amounts of these skin-healthy vitamins. Also, your doctor may recommend that you take a multivitamin to get extra amounts.

Indulge vices only in moderation. Research has shown that drinking alcohol can age the skin before its time. Smoking also causes problems because it constricts blood vessels in the skin, reducing the flow of oxygen. It's a good idea to limit your alcohol intake to a drink or two a day. If you smoke, of course, the sooner you can quit, the better it will be for your skin.

ABOUT THE AUTHOR

Brian Chichester is an award-winning health writer, licensed emergency medical technician, and certified personal trainer who follows many natural health care practices, including a rigorous exercise regimen. He has co-written several health books including *Powerfully Fit*, *Stress Blasters*, and *Sex Secrets* and has contributed articles to *Men's Health*, *Fitness*, *Tomorrow's Business Leader* and *Real Estate Today*. He is pursuing his master's degree in Public Health at the University of Glasgow, Scotland, on a competitive scholarship from Rotary International.